SOAR TO SUCCESS

Do Your Best on Nursing Tests!

D1444757

Paulette D. Rollant, PhD, MSN, RN, CCRN

President
Multi-Resources, Inc.
Newnan, Georgia

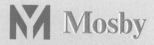 Mosby

St. Louis Baltimore Boston Carlsbad Chicago Minneapolis New York Philadelphia Portland
London Milan Sydney Tokyo Toronto

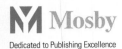
Dedicated to Publishing Excellence

Editor-in-Chief: Sally Schrefer
Senior Editor: Loren S. Wilson
Senior Developmental Editor: Brian Dennison
Project Manager: Deborah L. Vogel
Production Editor: Ed Alderman
Designer: Bill Drone

Composition by Top Graphics
Lithography/color film by R. R. Donnelley & Sons Company
Printing/binding by R. R. Donnelley & Sons Company

Mosby, Inc.
11830 Westline Industrial Drive
St. Louis, Missouri 63146

Library of Congress Cataloging-in-Publication Data
Rollant, Paulette D.
    Soar to success : do your best on nursing tests / Paulette D.
Rollant.
        p.   cm.
    Includes bibliographical references and index.
    ISBN 0-8151-3858-X (alk. paper)
    1. Nursing—Examinations, questions, etc.   2. Nursing—Study and
teaching.   I. Title.
    [DNLM: 1. Education, Nursing.   2. Educational Measurement nurses'
instruction.   3. Problem Solving nurses' instruction.   WY 18 R7455s
1999]
RT55.R653   1999
610.73'076—DC21
DNLM/DLC
for Library of Congress   99-10465
                                                                CIP

99   00   01   02   03   /   9   8   7   6   5   4   3   2   1

To Dan, my family, the students and graduates I have worked with over the years, and God who provides my faith, insight, talents, and abilities for success and happiness.

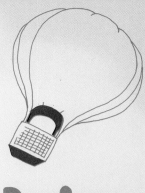

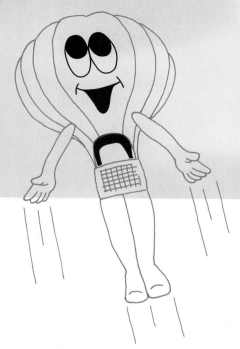

Preface

Do you study hard for tests only to find that, as a result, you have so much tension and fatigue that you can't even think?

Are you so concerned with the outcome of a test that you cannot concentrate on the process of tackling questions and using critical thinking?

Do you wish you had some practical strategies for diagnosing your test-taking errors and for implementing strategies to rise above them?

Would you appreciate some smart ways to improve your own guessing, for those moments (or those questions!) when that's really all you have going for you?

If you answered "yes," read on.

If you answered "yes" to even one of these questions, then consider this book your personal pilot's manual as you begin your journey through preparation for nursing exams. Based on my life experiences and academic knowledge, I have written this book for you.

Use this book as a navigational tool, not just in preparing for nursing board exams, but for everything from semester exams to unit tests in any course. Topics covered in this book include strategies for:

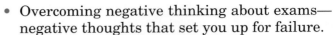

- Overcoming negative thinking about exams—negative thoughts that set you up for failure.
- Making the shift from outcome (grade-oriented) thinking to process (learning journey–oriented) thinking to relieve tension before it starts.
- Establishing a repertoire of physical and mental exercises that help you relax and unlock blocks in your thinking.
- Harnessing critical thinking as one of your best test-taking tools.
- Developing your own keys for memorizing and recall, especially through the use of storytelling and association.
- Acquiring specific, fun strategies for turning multiple-choice decisions into manageable, fun puzzles.
- Assessing, diagnosing, and "treating" your own testing errors.

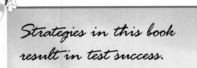

Strategies in this book result in test success.

As you scan the following chapters, start with what you think may be the most helpful to you. Remember to return to the evaluation checklists in Chapter 1 periodically and at the beginning of each quarter to reevaluate your progress. It is normal to have a variation in total scores (and sometimes, lower scores) at the beginning of the final quarter of school or before specific exams, such as licensing or certification. This simply reflects that you need to work harder to control your reactions to the exam situation.

I don't recommend reading this book in just one or two sittings. Think of it more as a handbook or a reference for when you are preparing for a test or reviewing test results.

Use this book as a handbook or reference.

- Flip through the chapters.
- Find something that catches your eye. Spend as much time there as you want or as you have available.

Sometimes small bits of information are more easily absorbed and recalled than larger chunks of content. Remember that it's the little things in life that make the difference.

I hope that by using this book (or even just referring to the parts that you feel apply specifically to you) you will be able to avoid the same negative thoughts and actions that I struggled with while taking tests during my 19 years of higher education (specifically, nursing education). Please benefit from my work as both a student and a teacher, adopting the test strategies specifically for nurses' exams offered in this book so that you can sail through test-taking from now on.

Preparing for and taking tests is a little bit like learning to fly a hot air balloon. You need the right equipment, the right attitude, and the right training. You need to know how to take advantage of those moments when the wind is blowing your way and what to do when it isn't. Take advantage of the air currents as they occur at each moment of your day.

Both balloon travel and test preparation require a checklist of your physical, intellectual, and emotional abilities for each and every event. The preparation checklist would include these items:

Physical

- Wear appropriate clothing.
- Eat before the trip.
- Pack a snack for delays.
- Pack for potential physical discomforts (such as remedies for headaches or gastrointestinal upset or saline solution for your dry eyes).
- Plan to rest before the test or trip so you can do your best and get enjoyment from the completion of the event.

Intellectual

- Think of what you "must" complete versus what you "want or would like" to complete before the event.
- Focus on the task at hand. Put all else aside.

The preparation checklist:
- *Physical*
- *Intellectual*
- *Emotional*

- Think of the positive aspects instead of the negative aspects. (For example, "I know some things and will be able to figure out the rest.")
- Learn to have fun; turn the events into fun puzzles.
- Focus on the steps in the process rather than only on the outcome of the event.

Emotional

- Tell yourself that you deserve this test or trip. You have worked hard in preparation for either event.
- Focus on the good feelings you are experiencing inside.
- Have an attitude of preparedness, an anticipation that nothing will happen that you can't control or work through so that your concentration can be maintained.
- Act happy—you will be happy.
- Think and act as if you will make lemonade out of the lemons thrown your way.

Practice, practice, practice—both mentally and physically—before a test just as you would before a hot air balloon trip. Practice may not make you perfect, but it will get the job done using the best of your abilities.

Test questions, answers and rationales, and test-taking tips are included in this book in Appendix B. Use these questions for your practice to further develop your skills in assessing, diagnosing, treating, and evaluating your own testing errors and abilities. Beware: Many of these questions are the higher level questions. They are designed to mold you into harnessing your critical thinking skills.

In summary, consider this book as your personal pilot's manual as you begin your journey through preparation for nursing exams. Use this book as a navigational tool, not just in preparing for nursing

Over 150 questions with answers, rationales, and test tips.

board exams, but for everything from quizzes to final exams in any course. Finally, use the strategies and advice in this book to:

- Balance your life between professional, family, and personal needs.
- Learn to seize the moment for your success.

Learn to seize the moment for your success.

ACKNOWLEDGMENTS

I express my deepest gratitude to those who have worked with me to make this book a reality. I have now "put into print" those helpful hints that, over the years, students and graduates have encouraged me to publish so that others can perform at their peak on tests.

I especially want to thank the following people:

From the early years:

Suzi Epstein, who began with me the idea and skeleton of this book; Jerry Schwartz, who also worked with me on the beginnings of the book; and Beverly Copland and Laurie Muench, who talked over ideas for this book while we worked on the Nursing Review Series.

From the past year:

Brian Dennison, my Senior Developmental Editor, who has the patience of Job and the skills of an expert negotiator when changes were needed, and who gave me much thoughtfulness and guidance to help me set priorities during all phases of publication. Thanks, Brian!

Also, Loren Wilson, who provided a global picture of publication needs; Ellen Stevens, Nichole Ambrosio, Lori Antezzo, and Barrie Quappe, the student reviewers; Mary E. Hanson-Zalot, RN, MSN, OCN, of Northeastern Hospital School of Nursing, who reviewed Appendix B, the practice test; Gary Clark, who did the balloon man illustrations; Don O'Conner, who did all the other illustrations; Bill Drone, the designer; Ed Alderman, the production editor; and Linda Wendling, the freelance editor.

Finally, Patricia Romick, MS, RNCS, Assistant Professor and Academic Counselor/Student Life Educator at the University of Texas School of Nursing at Galveston, who wrote Chapter 12, Psychosynthesis: Be a Star Test-Taker.

From over the years:

Dan, my husband of over 25 years, for his patience, humor, support, and love. His faith in my abilities has sustained my energies and maintained my sense of the priorities in life.

My parents, Joseph and Mildred Demaske, for their love. I especially thank Mom for her encouragement and prayers.

My brothers, Joe and Alan; my sisters, Joanne and Amy; and my sister-in-law, Amy Nemeth, who all encouraged me at the lowest moments.

My niece and godchild, Alana, for her bright smile and belly laugh that always brought me back to the real meaning of life: People are more important than papers. Thanks, Alana, for reminding me to take time to play!

Paulette D. Rollant

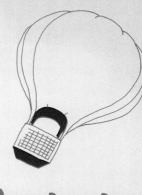

Contents

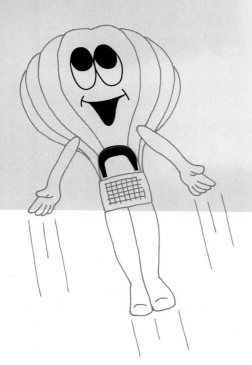

Appendixes

SOAR TO SUCCESS
Do Your Best on Nursing Tests!

An Invitation for New Ways to Prep for Tests: A Hot Air Balloon Trip

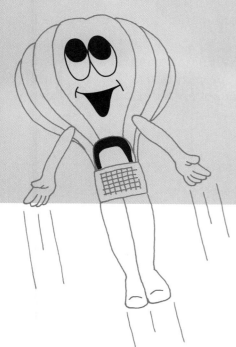

"You need to say to yourself, 'When you see me, you see a winner. I am who I say I am.' What you say in your mouth you believe in your heart."

Rosey Grier

Imagine that you have accepted an invitation to go for a hot air balloon ride. In preparation for this flight you may have many concerns or questions, such as the following:

- Am I afraid of heights?
- Should I even go?
- Who will be the pilot?
- Should I eat before the flight?
- What time of day will the flight take place?

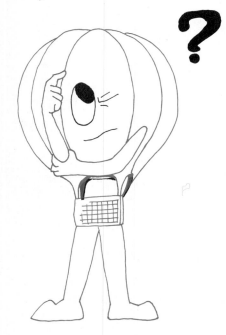

- What should I wear?
- Should I take a camera? Will I see my house?
- How many people will be in the basket?
- Do I need to read about ballooning before I go?
- How do I handle my nervousness to be able to enjoy the flight?

These are all practical questions and include, to some extent, a mental self-assessment. What should you do? To further explore what your attitude is about this opportunity, you might consider the following issues:

- How you think and feel about this type of flight
- The pros and cons of this chance to look at your environment from a new and somewhat scary angle
- What physical and mental preparation is necessary

Now I want you to think of using this book as a new experience for test preparation as you would use the new experience of a hot air balloon ride for viewing your home and city.

ARE YOU READY? SELF-ASSESSMENT

As a first step, it is critical for you to do a self-assessment of your thoughts and feelings toward tests and studying. If you think this self-assessment is unnecessary, ask yourself this: are you afraid to venture into unknown territory? Sometimes the results of self-assessment validate that personal thinking patterns, perceptions, or behaviors are the problem rather than external events or issues. If you avoid self-assessment, you are probably in the group of people who would turn down the opportunity to

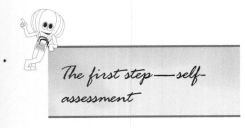

The first step—self-assessment

see familiar land from a balloon flight—a chance to learn more or change your perception about your home and city.

Keep in mind that without self-assessment you will not get the full benefit from this book in terms of improving your test preparation and test-taking skills. Recall the nursing process: assessment is the initial step in any situation. So start with self-assessment. Complete the Test Attitude Assessment (TAA) at the end of this chapter. You may periodically need to repeat the Test Attitude Assessment for a determination of new needs and a validation of changes in your behaviors.

GET ON YOUR MARK: PHYSICAL AND MENTAL PREPARATION

Physical and mental preparation are essential for the achievement of any goal. Many champion sports figures repeatedly talk about how they exercise physically every day and also prepare mentally for weekly or playoff games. You've heard them say, "I've mentally lost my edge." Or, "I'm in a slump and have to work on my attitude. I have to see myself hitting the ball."

The next time you watch a basketball player preparing for a foul shot, or a baseball player at bat, notice the following:

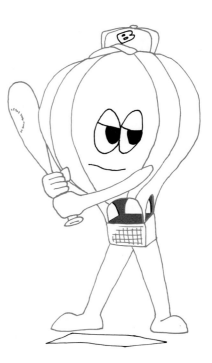

- The repetition of physical movements
- The mental concentration
- The intense focus of the eyes

Think of yourself as an athlete in your chosen area of study. How do you prepare for your tests? Is this preparation physical *and* mental?

Test preparation requires both physical and mental exercises. The physical actions might include the following:

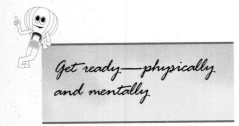

Get ready—physically and mentally

- Doing practice tests
- Reviewing how you read or look at the test questions and options
- Paying attention to body sensations before and during the test
- Attending class regularly

The mental actions might include the following:

- Having confidence in your study habits
- Countering negative comments or thoughts with positive affirmations
- Using various approaches to deal with stress before and during tests
- Thinking of pleasant things before a test

Make a list of your own physical and mental actions before and during tests. Now identify which of the behaviors you've listed that are positive or negative influences on your goal of doing your best on tests. Put a plus or minus sign next to each behavior in the list.

Now take a few minutes to compare your answers with the inventories of "Get on Your Mark" test behaviors found in Boxes 1-1 and 1-2. Then compare your behaviors list with the lists compiled by your friends. Learn from one another.

Check your behaviors
- *Before tests*
- *During tests*
- *After tests*

Box 1-1

Inventory of Physical
"Get on Your Mark" Test Behaviors

Directions: Check all behaviors that you currently use during test preparation or test-taking. Add any others that you use to this list.

☐ Get a good night's sleep before the exam.
☐ Eat a meal or snack 2 to 3 hours prior to the exam.
☐ Review my notes at least three times before the exam.
☐ Cram the night before if I haven't had time to study.
☐ Go for a walk or exercise before I study.
☐ Stretch my arms and legs at my seat before, during, and after the exam.
☐ Stop and periodically take some slow deep breaths.
☐ Do not study the night before an exam. Review any notes one time the day before. Do something fun the night before. (This helps reduce stressed feelings and reinforces feelings of preparedness.)
☐ Reward myself after the exam. Decide on a small gift or reward prior to studying for the exam. (This gives me something positive to look forward to after the exam.)
☐ Apply information to real people or experiences.

_____

_____

_____

_____

> **Box 1-2**

> ### *Inventory of Mental "Get on Your Mark" Test Behaviors*
>
> Directions: Check all the behaviors that you currently use during test preparation or test-taking. Add others that you use to the list.
>
> ☐ I think of all that I studied so that I don't forget it on the way to the exam.
> ☐ I keep repeating certain information to myself so that I don't forget it.
> ☐ I tell myself that I have studied enough and am prepared for the exam, and that I will not second-guess myself.
> ☐ I tell myself that I wish I had studied more.
> ☐ I tell myself the answer is there on the page or screen, I just need to identify it.
> ☐ I close my eyes and picture what is being said during lectures.
> ☐ I close my eyes and picture what is being asked on a question.
>
> _____
>
> _____
>
> _____
>
> _____

GET SET! SELECT NEW ACTIONS OR BEHAVIORS

After assessing your test attitudes and reflecting on your behaviors, develop new behaviors for test success. Use the following items as markers to guide you on your trip to a new source of test-taking success:

1. Select new actions or behaviors for test success as you read this book. The worksheet for the development of "Get on Your Mark" Actions found

Box 1-3

Worksheet for the Development of "Get on Your Mark" Actions

Directions:

1. Indicate the quarter/semester in which you did the self-assessment. Write this in terms of the month and the year.
2. Write in your score from the Test Attitude Assessment under TAA Total Score.
3. Look at the list of actions in Table 1-1 and select the physical and mental actions that might work for you. Select the necessary number of physical and mental actions as identified in the Interpretation of the Test Attitude Assessment Score.
4. Use these actions daily and before or during testing situations.
5. At the beginning of a new quarter or semester, cross out those actions that did not work for you. Add new actions.
6. Repeat this evaluation at the beginning of each quarter.

Quarter (Month/Year)	TAA Total Score	Physical "Get on Your Mark" Actions	Mental "Get on Your Mark" Actions
		1.	1.
		2.	2.
		3.	3.
		4.	4.

in Box 1-3 will help you select new behaviors that are useful to you.

2. Use these actions or behaviors on a daily basis so they become second nature to you.
3. Continue to apply them in study, review, and testing situations.

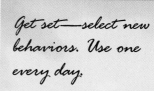

Get set—select new behaviors. Use one every day.

Table 1-1 "Get on Your Mark" Actions	
Physical Actions	**Mental Actions**
Go to bed early.	Say "no" more often.
Avoid tight clothes.	Identify difficult tasks; do these first.
Write things down.	Look at problems as challenges.
Avoid or minimize contact with negative people.	Look at problems as opportunities to grow.
Stretch.	Look for the silver lining or the good in any person or situation.
Breathe slowly and deeply.	Be aware of your decisions.
Dance to your favorite music.	Believe in yourself.
Whistle a tune.	Visualize the positive; visualize winning.
Pet an animal (dog, cat, snake, or hamster).	Develop a sense of humor.
Do it today; avoid procrastination.	Don't take yourself so seriously.
Maintain your weight.	Concentrate on the present, the "here and now."
Do things in moderation.	Stop thinking tomorrow will be better.
Stop and smell a flower.	Have a plan B and a plan C.
Find a "vent partner," someone who will listen without comment.	Identify your limits.
Talk less and listen more.	Remember that stress is an attitude.
Get to class early.	Share a big grin or smile with a stranger or someone you love.
Keep a journal.	Quit trying to fix others or situations.
Drive a different route to school or work.	Strive for achievement, not for perfection—it has to get done, it doesn't have to be perfect.
Get to work or school early.	Be aware that thoughts of being perfect perpetuate procrastination.
Play with a child (preschooler or toddler).	Get focused.
Do something new.	

4. In addition, use these actions during daily stressful events that are unrelated to testing or study.
5. Remember to select actions or behaviors that take the least amount of time (in general, 15 to 30 seconds) to use during a test.

You may want to repeat this chapter at the beginning of each quarter, semester, or prior to a major test. As your life events and experience change, so may your behaviors and your attitudes about tests.

Caution! As you near graduation and licensing/certification exams, your attitude may become either less anxious or more anxious. Only your continued self-assessment of behaviors and thoughts, coupled with interventions and evaluation, will keep you growing and improving!

SUMMARY

Completing the Test Attitude Assessment should tell you how many and what type of behaviors you need to start with to develop new ways to prepare for tests. Refer to chapters 4 and 5 for more specific exercises.

A high score on the Test Attitude Assessment indicates a high risk for making testing errors during exams—especially those exams considered to be major tests. A low score on the Test Attitude Assessment indicates a lower risk of testing errors. But beware! A lower score doesn't exempt you from testing errors. Sometimes persons with low scores on the Test Attitude Assessment have testing error behaviors so ingrained that they repeatedly make the wrong choices in actual test situations despite their favorable assessment scores.

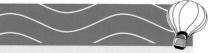

Go! You're on the way to test success.

Air Currents

"Either you let your life slip away by not doing the things you want to, or you get up and do them."

Carl Ally

TEST ATTITUDE ASSESSMENT

Directions: Read each statement; then respond by circling either "yes" or "no." Base your answers on how you generally feel before, during, and after tests. There are no right or wrong answers. Do not spend too much time on any one statement, but give the answer that seems to best describe how you generally feel.

Physiological Reactions

During major tests:

Yes No While taking exams, I have an uneasy, upset feeling.

Yes No I shake my foot or leg rapidly.

Yes No I feel impatient and jumpy.

Yes No I can feel my heart race from time to time.

Yes No I am so tense that my stomach gets upset.

Yes No I have difficulty staying awake and alert.

Yes No I feel very anxious.

Yes No I feel panicky when I take tests on a computer.

Yes No I feel my heart beating very fast.

Yes No I have feelings of being physically drained, washed out, or exhausted.

Yes No I get mild to severe headaches or have blurred vision.

Yes No I feel myself getting more anxious and less able to concentrate as others finish their tests.

Yes   No   I see words that are not there or that are similar to the given words.

Yes   No   I have to stop for bathroom breaks every few minutes.

Yes   No   I give up trying to concentrate after 1 to 1½ hours of testing because I become tired.

Mental Reactions

Just before a major test:

Yes   No   I rarely feel self-assured, calm, and optimistic.

Yes   No   I have an unpleasant, troubled feeling.

Yes   No   I draw a blank.

Yes   No   I find myself worrying about the consequences of failing.

Yes   No   Although I think I know the content well, I fear that the test will cover content that I have not studied.

During a major test:

Yes   No   I think about my failing the test, and this interferes with my performance.

Yes   No   I draw frequent blanks at the beginning of or during the test.

Yes   No   I find myself thinking about whether I'll ever get finished with the test.

Yes   No   I get more puzzled as I work harder at trying to think clearly.

Yes   No   I have perceptions of doing poorly, and this interferes with my attention to details on the test.

Yes No I feel there is content that I have not studied, although I think I know the content well.

Yes No I seem to disappoint myself while working on the harder test questions.

Yes No I am bothered mentally, which causes physical discomforts.

Yes No I find myself worrying about the consequences of failing.

Yes No I often feel that my mind freezes, making me forget content I know.

Yes No I feel nervous when thinking about getting my test results back.

Yes No I worry about how well I've scored on an exam compared with others.

Yes No My scores on practice tests interfere with my work on tests.

Yes No During exams I find myself thinking about whether I'll ever make it.

Yes No I know I spend too much time on some questions, but I can't stop this.

INTERPRETATION OF THE TEST ATTITUDE ASSESSMENT SCORE

1. My score (total number of yes answers) is _____.

2. This means that I need to practice at least (see reference on p. 13):

   _____ physical behaviors to prepare for or use during a test.

   _____ mental behaviors to prepare for or use during a test.

If you have 10 or less "yes" answers, practice at least one physical and one mental behavior for testing every other day.

If you have more than 10 but less than 20 "yes" answers, practice at least two physical and two mental behaviors for testing every day.

If you have more than 20 but less than 30 "yes" answers, practice at least three physical and three mental behaviors for testing. Practice them twice a day.

If you have 30 or more "yes" answers, practice at least four physical and four mental behaviors for testing. Practice them three times a day.

Choosing Balloons: Two Types of Thinking

"The rainbows of the mind brighten the skies of our life with color, grace, and contrast against stormy clouds."

Joyce Wycoff

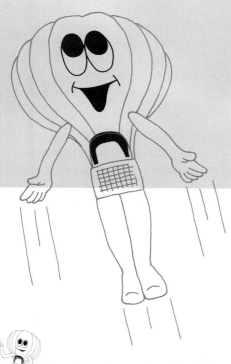

Choose the right type of thinking: process over outcome.

The balloon is just one type of airship. The type of airship you fly will, of course, greatly affect your trip. Similarly, different types of thinking can either hinder or help you on tests, through your nursing program, and throughout your life. Selecting the right type of thinking can make all the difference.

Two types of thinking work together to ultimately provide balance in anyone's life: outcome thinking and process thinking. *Outcome thinking* is narrowly focused on deliberate, specific results. For example, "I need (want) (have) to make all A's throughout school."

Process thinking is more broadly based with general thoughts for a wider range of acceptable results.

15

Process thinking is also more concerned with the whole learning "journey" or experience. For example, "I will graduate in a timely manner as influenced by my family's activities or other life events." The use of both types of thinking includes the mental use of little steps that result in big changes for a balanced, more enjoyable life.

Do your goals focus on making certain grades? On reaching graduation day? Do you give little or no consideration to:

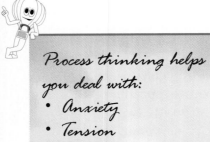

- The number of classes taken?
  - Events taking place in your home or social life?
  - The number of roles you take on each day?
  - How you are changing as you go through your education program?
  - How your friends or family members are changing as you go through your education program?

If you answered "yes" to most of these questions, then your one focus—to graduate—is an *outcome* focus, with grades and graduation seen as a *product*. This approach is unbalanced and one-sided. It *fails to look at the process toward* graduation (the type and sequencing of actions for the achievement of a more specific learning goal). Using this approach will place you in danger of not performing at maximum effectiveness and efficiency!

MY STRUGGLE TO OVERCOME OUTCOME THINKING

Process thinking helps you deal with:
- *Anxiety*
- *Tension*
- *Fatigue*

I, too, was an outcome-focused student for many of the years it took to complete my nursing education. (It took 19 years, to be exact: 3 years for the nursing diploma, 7 years for the BSN, 2 years for the MSN, and 7 years for the PhD.) I kept going back to school, not because I loved to study, but because I was always one academic degree short for either keeping my current job or qualifying for my next job.

I had a long history of outcome-focused thinking even before that, though. I set an internal measuring stick or goal for myself years ago in the primary grades, telling myself that I had to make the highest grades. I constantly struggled with the mind-set that a grade of 98% wasn't good enough; I had to make 100%. I felt bad if I didn't make the highest grade in the class or make 100%. I looked at what was wrong with the test questions rather than at my behaviors. In fact, I never examined my negative and positive behaviors toward preparing for and taking tests.

At some point during my educational process, I realized that the outcome of consistently achieving the highest grades had eluded me. And then, after 10 years of working as a competent, knowledgeable registered nurse, I had a major failure. I completed the course work for my master's degree, but I failed the exit exam. It was 6 months before I could retake the exam. By not having the degree in hand, I lost both the salary and the title that I had negotiated in my new job. The good news, at least, was that I did still have the job.

Only then did I force myself to look at the behaviors I relied on in studying for and taking exams. I knew the content, yet I couldn't apply my knowledge during tests! When I got my test back I saw that sometimes I marked the wrong answer when I knew the correct answer. I had no idea why this happened.

After this major failure, I forced myself to look at the way my mind and body responded to anxiety, tension, and fatigue. I also looked at my actions in dealing with these feelings—not just in testing situations, but in my life events as well. This was the first step in my using *process* thinking.

Before this failure, I had the perception that people who did relaxation, imagery, and similar exercises were people with bigger problems than mine. After my major failure, I *finally* accepted that *I had a problem* with controlling my anxiety, tension, and fatigue in

"Learn to think; then study and renew."
Paulette Rollant

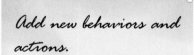

Add new behaviors and actions.

Add stress coping resources: improve your performance!

different situations. I saw that I used many negative behaviors, including denial, in response to these sensations, especially during tests. These negative behaviors affected my ability to demonstrate what I knew! I finally accepted that I needed to add new behaviors and actions. This included new mental and physical activities aimed at identifying times when I was anxious, tense, or tired, and other new behaviors and actions to bring these feelings within a controllable level before and during tests.

During the 5 months leading up to the repeat exam I did some self-study and started to do some relaxation and imagery exercises. This time I was successful in passing and did graduate with my master's degree.

Years later I took a stress management course as one of the first courses in my doctoral studies. This course planted a seed that blossomed into the research focus for my dissertation: stress coping resource development in beginning nursing students. My research involved studying three groups of students during one quarter. The results reflected that the students who routinely practiced some type of action aimed at reducing tension or fatigue had overall improved performance during that quarter.

Now I strongly believe in and daily perform at least two or three relaxation exercises. I usually start with a 1-mile walk, during which I constantly replace any negative thoughts that pop into my mind with positive ones. As I walk and think, I enjoy the nature around me.

Every 2 to 3 hours throughout the day, I do a neck muscle check, looking for tightness. I usually have to do neck and shoulder tightening/loosening exercises at these check times. I also think of what has happened in the past 3 hours that might cause me to be tense or tired.

At night when I first get into bed, I close my eyes and do a head-to-toe body scan. I achieve relaxed muscles from head to toe. Afterwards, I repeat at least eight to ten times a positive thought to end my day (for example, "I am doing better at improving my patience"). When I was in school I repeated to myself things like: "I am getting better at identifying key words in the test questions"; or, "I feel more relaxed after the tense/relax muscle exercises"; or, "I am improving at my behaviors during tests. I had nausea only once during today's test instead of my usual four times."

Shift your focus from outcome to process.

HOW TO RISE ABOVE OUTCOME THINKING

What, then, might be a first step in rising above the outcome-focused way of thinking? Try this: Simply look up. Look away from the outcome. Unleash your creativity, imagination, and enthusiasm for different actions. Focusing on the processes of thinking and of restoring balance in your study time can lead to the following:

Find a phrase that puts wind into your sails.

- Better problem solving
- Better use of your time
- More enjoyment of your family
- More fun time for yourself

When is the last time you said to yourself, "I love living!" Or, "I have some fun each day of my life!" Or, "Life is G-R-R-EAT!" Did you say these statements out loud and with enthusiasm? Or did you just think them as dull thoughts?

Come up with a phrase that puts the wind back into your sails. I developed the following phrase as I struggled with attempts to balance the demands of school with everything else in my life: "People are more important than papers." I used it as my rule to reel me in when I drifted aimlessly; became anxious, tense, or tired; or when I became unbalanced by having school as the only focus in my life.

This was my phrase. Then I paired it with actions

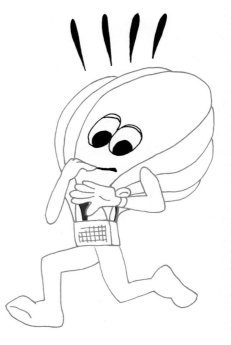

Consistently take time for those you love— people are more important than papers.

to balance, deal with, and prevent school stress. Sundays were set aside for my husband, Dan, and me or for other family events. At times, with self-induced pressure to have certain outcomes, I had anxiety about sticking to this rule. However, I countered such feelings with these thoughts: "I can find other time to do that specific school work. I'll get up early or stay up late one of the other 6 days in the week." Or, "Pleasant memories of people will mean more to me long after the people are gone." Or, "People *are* more important than papers." So, no matter what, I stuck to it for over 7 years! And I graduated! You can too!

So take that scheduled 30 minutes or that entire weekend and give full attention to the people you love and care about. Take time for family and friends, and do it consistently. You won't regret it.

HOW TO DEVELOP PROCESS THINKING

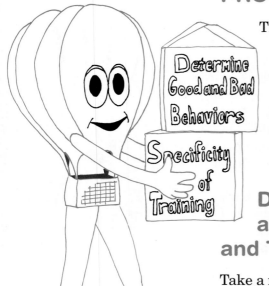

There are two activities that can help you develop your process thinking abilities: (1) determining your bad and good behaviors, and (2) specificity of training. Both require consistent action and follow-up. Once you determine which behaviors have the best results, your test preparation and test-taking performance will begin to improve.

Determining Good and Bad Learning and Testing Behaviors

Take a moment to reflect on the process part of being in school. What are your bad and good behaviors when you study and take tests? I'll give you some examples of each to get you started thinking. Table 2-1 is a list of good and bad learning behaviors. Table 2-2 presents testing behaviors. Circle those behaviors that remind you of your own study and test-taking habits. Add any additional behaviors to the bottom of each list.

Bad actions? I have used the word "bad" rather than "behavior for improvement" because I believe these behaviors really are bad and detrimental to your overall performance. It's like a weak piece of wood holding up a wooden deck. Sooner of later it results in a deck that falls either partially or totally. The fall will be unexpected and without warning. The same process can happen with your persistent use of bad behaviors. Bad behaviors drain your ability to do your best. Then one day, without warning, you'll find yourself in a major crisis on a major test.

Now that you have a clearer idea of these study behaviors, what should you do? Take one small bad behavior and substitute one good behavior for it. Repeat this substitution daily for 1 week. The next week, exchange a second bad behavior for a second appropriate substitute. You will notice changes such as the following:

- Your attitude will be more positive.
- Your sense of accomplishment will grow with the knowledge that you are getting things done or have made some improvement.
- You will find that you actually have more time for yourself!

Continue in this manner if you find these good behaviors helpful. Practice them for a whole month. By then they should turn into your mode of persistent, positive actions.

Are you not sure about where to begin? Are you overwhelmed in selecting where to start? Consider looking at the amount of stress you have that is caused by time management. Many people struggle with the perception of not having enough time. They

Identify good and bad testing-study behaviors so that you know what to change and when to change it.

Substitute a good behavior for a bad behavior—a week or a month at a time—until each one becomes a habit.

Table 2-1   Learning Behaviors

Physical Behaviors		Mental Behaviors	
Good	**Bad**	**Good**	**Bad**
I have a daily time set aside to study.	I study only a day or two before the test.	I select background music based on the type of content I will be reviewing.	I keep feeling bad—I plan to change my study habits, but I never have the time.
I study at a consistent time.	I rarely read the text.	I review with friends for no longer than 1½-2 hours, and we stick to the point.	I think that daily things that pop up are more important, so I wait until the last minute to study.
I have a daily time set aside for myself to play.	I study only my notes.	I have mental breaks every 45-50 minutes when I study.	I think to study only my notes most of the time.
I read the chapter summary before the class covering that content.	I review with friends, and we talk more than study.	I take mental breaks when I feel tired or tense while studying.	During my study time, I keep having flashbacks of how poorly I have done on prior tests from this instructor or in this course.
I use review texts or cards to study.	I study with any kind of noise (TV, radio on, noisy house).	I tell myself I won't know everything.	I tell myself I'll need to remember all of the material covered to pass the test.
I study with specific music in the background.	I study so intensely that I keep the same position for hours as I study.	Add your own:	Add your own:
I change my study location from time to time and limit it to two or three consistent places.	I never change my study location.		
Add your own:	Add your own:		

Table 2-2   Testing Behaviors

Physical Behaviors		Mental Behaviors	
Good	**Bad**	**Good**	**Bad**
I eat on the morning before an exam. I limit my caffeinated fluids before exams. I keep plugging away on a test no matter how tired I am. When I'm scared I change my position in the chair during a test. I get enough rest the night before a test. Add your own:	I don't eat on the morning before an exam. I eat junk food before exams. I drink a lot of caffeinated fluids before exams (coffee, tea, soda, or chocolate). I stay up late the night before a test. Add your own:	I tell myself I am ready for the test. I keep plugging away on a test no matter how tired I am. When I'm scared I take time to change my thoughts during a test. I tell myself I am rested and ready the morning of a test. I tell myself the answer is on the page or screen. I just have to find it. Add your own:	I think of what I didn't study and what I don't know while on the way to the exam. I give up sometimes after the first few questions or toward the end of the exam, especially if it is long. I expect to know about *all* the content on a test. Add your own:

rush and panic rather than take the time to see how outcome thinking creates this behavior—and creates stress. They blame family, circumstances, or schedules for robbing them of time. Does this sound familiar?

If so, this is a good place to start to change your thinking. Change your goal. Instead of trying to be so organized that you get everything done and have more free time (outcome thinking), try to be able to feel that it is okay not to be able to get everything

> "Small hinges swing large doors."
> W. Clement Stone

done but to accept things as they are (process thinking). It's okay to have 10 minutes of free time instead of 2 hours of free time.

Specificity of Training

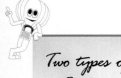

Specificity of training: to be better at studying and testing, practice studying and test questions every day.

When we began to explore ways to develop process thinking, we also mentioned specificity of training as the other side of changing bad behaviors. What is specificity of training? There is a rule in exercise science: if you want to become a better distance runner, practice distance running. This is called *specificity of training*. To be a better test-taker, practice answering test questions. If you want to be better at studying, set aside time every day to study. Discipline, consistency, and persistence are keys for unlocking the door of change. Get to know your pattern of errors in thinking, reading, perceiving, interpreting, doubting, selecting, defining, formulating, and recalling before and during tests. Then substitute new actions that will help you to become more efficient and effective in testing. Who knows? You may even have time left over to have fun!

Three keys:
- *Discipline*
- *Consistency*
- *Persistence*

SUMMARY

Recall the two types of thinking. Outcome thinking is more narrowly focused on deliberate, specific, rigid results. For example, "I need (want) (have) to make all A's throughout school." Process thinking is more broadly based on general thoughts with a wider range of acceptable results. It takes into consideration other aspects of living and the whole learning experience. For example, "I will graduate in a timely manner as influenced by my family's activities or other life events." The use of both types of thinking includes the mental use of little steps that result in big changes for a balanced, more enjoyable life.

Two types of thinking:
- *Outcome*
- *Process*

Air Currents

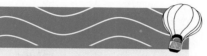

"Remember the two benefits of failure:

- *If you do fail, you learn what doesn't work.*
- *The failure gives you an opportunity to do a new approach."*

Roger von Oech

"Children enter school as question marks and leave as periods."

Neil Postman

"The greatest discovery of my generation is that a human being can alter his life by altering his attitude."

William James

Get Ready for Test Success: The Four Cs and Five HTs

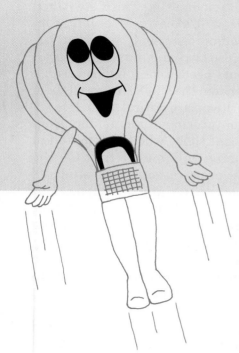

"Some painters transform the sun into a yellow spot; others transform a yellow spot into the sun."

Pablo Picasso

So far, we've touched on ways to evaluate your own study techniques and ways to shift from outcome thinking to process thinking. In the next chapter, we'll begin steps toward piloting your thinking. But before beginning even a practice flight, a pilot must check the equipment to be sure he or she has—or knows where to find—everything needed for a successful journey. In the same way, preparing for a test involves making sure one is equipped for the journey.

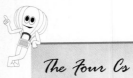

The Four Cs of test success:

1. Content

2. Control

3. Confidence

4. Common sense

CHECKING YOUR FOUR Cs BEFORE TAKING OFF

Before beginning any flight, a hot air balloon pilot needs to have four key factors in place. First, of course, all equipment—the basic *content* of the airship—must be in place. Related to this, the pilot needs to be sure—before leaving the ground—that he or she will have *control* once the balloon is airborne. And finally, no one wants to fly unless the pilot has both *confidence* and *common sense*! These same four factors—termed the Four Cs—can be applied to test preparation. Tips for implementing these are called the Five HTs, or the "How To's" of using content, control, confidence, and common sense.

These Four Cs can also be compared to the four essential physical elements needed for a balloon trip: a balloon, a basket, hot air, and the wind. Not one of them can be ignored. All four items are critical to success.

In my experience of tutoring students and graduates, I have noticed that those who fail tend to fall into the habit of focusing only on the first C—the content needed for test preparation. These students know the content backwards and forwards. But when their minds block or freeze up during a test, they have no confidence in the use of test-taking strategies and little or no control over the tension or fatigue that occurs during the test. This leaves them unable to use common sense. Let me stress again that all four elements are necessary for consistent, successful performance on tests.

Let's compare the structure and mechanism of a hot air balloon flight to the Four Cs for test preparation. (See Figure 3-1 for an illustration of this comparison.)

Content

The balloon can be likened to the content you need to carry with you into a test. Let's look at a hot air

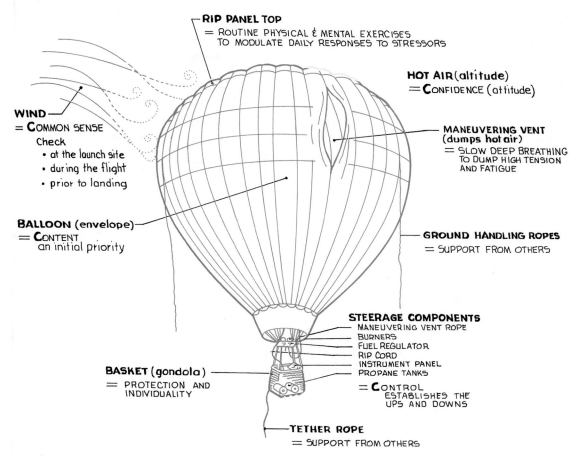

RIP PANEL TOP
= ROUTINE PHYSICAL & MENTAL EXERCISES TO MODULATE DAILY RESPONSES TO STRESSORS

HOT AIR (altitude)
= **C**ONFIDENCE (attitude)

WIND
= **C**OMMON SENSE
Check
• at the launch site
• during the flight
• prior to landing

MANEUVERING VENT (dumps hot air)
= SLOW DEEP BREATHING TO DUMP HIGH TENSION AND FATIGUE

BALLOON (envelope)
= **C**ONTENT
an initial priority

GROUND HANDLING ROPES
= SUPPORT FROM OTHERS

STEERAGE COMPONENTS
MANEUVERING VENT ROPE
BURNERS
FUEL REGULATOR
RIP CORD
INSTRUMENT PANEL
PROPANE TANKS
= **C**ONTROL ESTABLISHES THE UPS AND DOWNS

BASKET (gondola)
= PROTECTION AND INDIVIDUALITY

TETHER ROPE
= SUPPORT FROM OTHERS

Figure 3-1   The basic makeup of a hot air balloon and the Four Cs of test preparation.

balloon. It is made up of (1) the balloon and (2) the basket. The balloon and basket are connected by cables or ropes. Each balloon system is as individual as its owner, because the owner selects the size, color, and design that reflects his or her personality, likes, and dislikes. To get content into your memory and be able to recall it later (especially during times of stress) is the first priority for test preparation.

Similarly, each of you has unique knowledge, behaviors, thoughts, and feelings in a test situation. And

To get, then recall content is the initial priority for test preparation.

just like in ballooning, two items are essential for success in test situations: (1) content and (2) control.

Just as the balloon is connected to a basket by cables or ropes during the flight, your recall of content during a test is connected to control of yourself. This means that the smoothest possible sailing in any testing situation depends on certain simple, learned behaviors that can control tension and fatigue.

Before every balloon launch, the pilot makes a visual inspection of the following equipment: the balloon, the basket, the fuel system, and the instruments. The balloon's interior is examined for rips, for discolorations or changes in the heat-sensitive tabs, and for tangled vent ropes. Further preparations for flight are continued only after the system is inspected and found airworthy. Operators are also required to have this equipment inspected yearly by a government agency.

Similarly, an inspection is required before a test. Do you inspect your behaviors, thoughts, or feelings for wear and tear before and after each test? Do you do a check for not only *what,* but also *how* you have studied? Key areas for inspection should address these questions:

- When doing practice questions, do you consistently read the entire question and all the options?
- How do you deal with "mental blocks?"
- What are the most effective ways for you to recall content while studying? While doing practice questions? While taking the test?
- Do you enjoy learning or recalling content? Or is it an unpleasant chore?
- What actions do you think are vital before a test to feel prepared (ready for flight)? Or do you think you can never be prepared?

As with ballooning, routine checks of the whats and whys of content preparation for each test can better your chances of success and higher test scores.

> *"To know where you're going, and how to get there, you must first know yourself!"*
> W. Clement Stone

Control

A hot air balloon's controls, or steering mechanisms, can be compared to your control of your reactions and responses during a test. The balloonist makes sure all steering components are working properly. The fuel system, vent ropes, heat sensors, and guide ropes all contribute directly to controlling the altitude of the balloon. The basket also lends control by providing balance as it carries the pilot, passengers, navigation instruments, and fuel system. Most baskets have padded edges and thick leather scuff guards around their bottoms to protect them from damage if they are dragged sideways or tipped over. And so the basket serves as an alternative protective device when events don't go as planned in the phases of launching, ballooning, or landing, and it provides yet another element of control.

Control your fatigue and tension— externally and internally.

Similarly, the controls you have within can help you focus your attention, set priorities, and access recall. You can also adjust your reactions to uncontrollable external events and balance these by using your internal controls.

Do you have protective devices in place for test preparation and testing situations? What are your controls? Before or during a test are you aware of increasing:

- Tension?
- Fatigue?
- Despair?

What repetitive actions tend to lower your scores? Changing answers? Selecting options that you know nothing about? If you are aware of such damaging behaviors, do you do anything about them?

- Do you want to?
- Do you know how to?
- If you do change actions, are the new behaviors effective?

How are your exterior and interior—physical and mental aspects—protected? Have you been:

- Eating right?
- Getting some exercise?
- Getting enough rest?
- Spending any time with the family?
- Spending any time doing what you enjoy? (This is very important in establishing balance in your life, both for you and for your family.)

Do you reflect yearly about what patterns of test preparation and behaviors during tests you have developed or changed? Have you evaluated their effectiveness in terms of time, effort, and results?

One of the great dangers of being in school is in learning the right stuff without living by the right actions. Test-taking skills, like ballooning skills, require controls for a continuous balancing of internal and external events.

Confidence

The hot air in a balloon is similar to the confidence that you establish by acquiring effective skills: hot air establishes the altitude; confidence establishes your attitude.

The fuel system for a balloon usually consists of propane tanks and a burner mounted on a rack between the basket and the balloon. The pilot controls the burner, which produces hot air inside the balloon. Because this hot air is lighter than the surrounding air, the balloon rises and lifts the basket.

The hot air is typically released in a series of short bursts rather than in a long single burst. This allows time for the hot air to spread out in the balloon and prevents overheating the fabric.

By controlling the amount of hot air, the pilot controls the ascent and descent of the balloon (but not the flight pattern). The pilot, confident in the use of old and new skills, knows when to increase the intensity of the burner to create more hot air and make the balloon rise. The skilled pilot also senses when it is time to release hot air through the specially designed deflation ports or vents and lower the balloon's altitude. These types of decisions are grounded in prior knowledge or experience as well as updated knowledge and skills.

Your confidence establishes "what content" is being tested and "what about the content" is being asked.

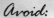

Check your confidence altitude—avoid both over- and under-confidence.

- Do you, like the balloon pilot, have confidence in your skills to read and evaluate the question? The stem (information given before the actual question)? All of the options?
- Do you take short cuts that lead to errors in reading and thinking?
- Do you use any specific processes to narrow the options to two? How do you decide between two options that both seem to answer the question?
- Do you ground your actions in prior knowledge and experiences and use updated knowledge and skills?
- Do you have confidence in yourself to regain your thinking skills after being rattled by a strange or extremely difficult test question?
- Do you use any confidence boosting affirmations during a test?
- Did you know that strategies exist to help increase your confidence to successfully take multiple choice tests?

Avoid:
- Short cuts when you read
- Random guessing
- Emotional decision-making

With confidence from the use of both old and new skills, you will know when to increase the intensity of your actions during a test. You will make judgments based on valid, effective reading skills, prior knowledge, and minimal emotional reactions.

Common sense, like the wind on a balloon, gives direction to decision-making.

Common Sense

The wind can be likened to your common sense. The strength and direction of the wind determines the course of flight for a hot air balloon; common sense lends direction to decision-making. Even though the pilot gets weather forecasting data prior to arrival at the launch site, the pilot continually evaluates weather conditions at decisive times, such as the following:

- At the launch site
- Just before lift off
- While in the air
- Just before landing

The pilot notes cloud types along with the direction in which trees sway and the way smoke rises. This helps the pilot determine actions that will produce a safe and enjoyable flight.

Your common sense establishes your attitude. Just as the events of the flight are out of the pilot's control, the test questions are out of your control. The following items can vary from test to test and from instructor to instructor:

- The types of questions
- The level of question difficulty
- The amount and type of wording
- The manner in which content is covered

But elements common to many test questions, like the common movements that balloon pilots use to determine a good flight, can alert you to the best answer. To use these common elements, you must apply your common sense.

On any given test, material unrelated to what you have studied will be found within some questions. If the material is unknown to you and you're having trouble selecting an option, what should you do? Simply use common sense. Ask yourself whether there may be a reason you don't understand these options. Look at the options in a different manner.

Use categories or themes under which you can place the options.

In summary, with a system similar to that needed for flight—a balloon, maneuvering equipment, hot air, and the wind (or content, control, confidence, and common sense)—you will soar to success and do well on tests! If one of the Four Cs is ignored or not practiced, your chances of consistent success on tests will be lower.

THE FIVE HTS: THE HOW TO'S OF CONTENT, CONTROL, CONFIDENCE, AND COMMON SENSE

HT Number One: The How To's of Content Prep—Eight Actions Before Course Tests

1. **Do something *every* day!**
   a. Review daily, for 10 to 15 minutes, some component of content for each class.
   b. Set your timer and limit yourself to get the most out of this 10 to 15 minutes!
   c. Then go on and do the same for any other class.
2. **Check your syllabus more than once!** Every week, before each of your classes, check the syllabus for chapters that will be covered. Use the following process to read each chapter. Read in this sequence:
   a. The introduction
   b. The major headings
   c. The chapter summaries of the chapters assigned that week

   Use this technique at one of your 15-minute study sessions. Check your syllabus before your classes to increase your listening skills and note-taking ability during the classes.
3. **Just listen!**

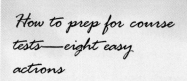

"A great mistake is doing nothing at all because you could do a little. Enough littles add up to a lot."

D. Aslett

How to prep for course tests—eight easy actions

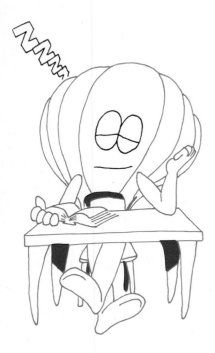

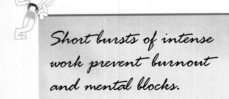

Short bursts of intense work prevent burnout and mental blocks.

- Go to class and listen.
- Close your eyes during the lecture and make an image in your mind of what is being said.
- Take notes only with a focus on major headings or topics followed only by details of information *unfamiliar* to you that you might need to look up later.

4. **Fall asleep on your books? Yes!**
   - Review for tests for 60 to 90 minutes, then relax. This may mean stretching, meditating, or taking a nap of at least 1½ to 2 hours.

5. **Review your notes just before bedtime.** This can increase your ability to retain the studied content as long-term memory. In some cases, reviewing before sleep has helped to improve recall of information for weeks rather than a few days.

6. **Limit your study time.** Study for no longer than 1 to 2 hours at a sitting! Recall that on a hot air balloon trip, the pilot uses short bursts of intense heat rather than a long burn for more effective rising and to prevent burning the balloon. These short bursts allow for the even spreading of the hot air in the balloon.

   Similarly, short bursts of study time allow for better cementing of any content into your memory. Avoid the trap of thinking that a marathon study session means learning more. This thought creates a false sense of security. Your aim is for effective study time, not for a long study time.

7. **Use associations to remember difficult content.** Is the content hard to remember? Try to identify it with something you find easy to relate to or understand. If it works for you, make up a story or think of a symbol. Associate the content with the story, the symbol, or something else familiar to you.

   For example, I once had difficulty recalling information about the liver. One day, as I prepared for a lecture on liver function, I got the idea to associate the liver's functions with the buildings found in any town or city. From that setup, I then associated serum tests of the liver with people's names who might work in each building. To recall some of the test values, I made up characteristics of the people and associated these with normal test values. Chapter 7 has more specific examples of the use of stories to take control of unruly content.

8. **Your best place to study is:**
   - Every place. Have productivity as a result of availability!
   - Portable. Have some type of study cards, text, or notes with you at all times. It's perfect (and fun) to catch inspiration that floats by sometimes when your mind is at rest or on something else.

HT Number Two: The How To's of Content Prep—Four Steps Before Comprehensive Tests

Different balloons need different preparations. Different balloons reflect different people, designs, and materials. It's a personal and individual thing. Well, different exams require different preparations. To prepare for those comprehensive/standardized/licensing exams, use the following four steps:

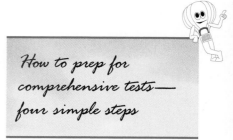

How to prep for comprehensive tests— four simple steps

1. **Purchase a good test review book.** Look for one that has the following essential characteristics:
   a. An outline of content that is
      - Easy to follow
      - Concise
      - Has items listed in order of priority
   b. Questions divided into content areas
   c. A format of simple multiple choice questions— the stem plus four options
   d. Answers with rationales and test tips
   e. Answers at the end of each section or test, rather than at the end of the book. This makes it easier and more efficient to use because less time is needed to look for the answers and rationales.

f. At least one 100-item test or at least one exam with the number of test items equal to the number of test items on your comprehensive/licensing exam.

2. **Sit down and answer a number of practice questions equal to the number of questions on your upcoming exam.** Have an answer sheet and three index cards with you at the time you take this practice exam. If possible, do this practice exam at the time of day when you are to take the real exam.

3. **Use three index cards.** As you finish the exam, immediately write down on the *first* index card:
   - At what part of the exam were you most tense? Or tired?
   - When was your thinking the best? At the beginning? The middle? Or at the end of the exam?
   - What influencing factors were present? Did you have any physical discomfort from what you ate or did prior to the exam? Crises at home? Illness? Did you do any physical or mental exercises before or during the exam? Did the exercises help? Put a smiley face ☺ next to the ones that helped you. Cross through any that were useless.

   Use the *second* index card when you correct your test. List the content or questions that you missed under the two categories of:
   - Could not recall or recognize
   - Knew, but missed somehow (maybe misread)

   On the *third* index card, group missed content under the organ systems (such as cardiac and neurologic) and the steps of the nursing process. This gives you a better idea of:
   - What organ systems or nursing process steps need more study
   - What areas on a test are most likely to make you more tense or tired

4. **Study and review.** Study the content listed under the "could not recall or recognize" label on the *second* index card. Look up this content in your review text or class text. Use your notes as a last resort

since comprehensive, standardized, or licensing exams are based on national content rather than local protocol. Then, if you have more time, review the other "knew but missed somehow" list. Look for patterns of misreading questions or options.

HT Number Three—The How To's of Tension and Fatigue Control

For test situations, just as for trips in a hot air balloon, it is essential for the pilot to control two factors:

- Tension
- Fatigue

If either factor becomes too much or uncontrollable, the situation becomes risky. The end results will be poor.

Think of yourself as the pilot of your reactions during the exam. You can control tension and fatigue to perform better on exams. Most people are tense at the beginning of an exam and tired at the end.

Both situations cause errors in judgment and difficulty in selecting the best option. With exams of more than 100 questions the fatigue factor sets in heavily, like a thick fog overcoming the brain's thinking ability. The most common reactions to this are either to read quickly or to skip over options to get the test over with sooner (or within the allotted time).

Evaluating Three Factors that Influence Tension and Fatigue

The following three factors influence the amount of tension and fatigue you have during exams:

1. Your life events of the prior day, week, month, or year

Evaluate three factors that influence your tension and fatigue.

2. Your health status
3. Your degree of satisfaction with your preparation

Take a look at Boxes 3-1, 3-2, and 3-3. As you read over each item, either answer the questions or place a check to the left of the statement if you have thought or acted in that manner. Next, reflect on whether your thoughts and behaviors are more inclined to be in a positive or negative trend. Then in the margin write one new approach to behavior or thinking that you will do daily within the next 2 weeks.

Box 3-1

Your Life Events of the Prior Day, Week, Month, or Year—How Did (Do) These Influence Your Abilities?

- Some events you have control over. For other events, you at least have control over your reactions/responses. Have you attempted to control *all* events in the past few weeks? Or have you attempted only to control your reaction or response to the events?
- Do you consistently tell yourself, "I will respond rather than react to life events?" In a response, the emotional lead takes a back seat and a combination of intellectual and emotional thinking takes the driver's seat.
- Don't discount your emotions! But do you practice putting them into their proper perspective? If feelings controlled people's ability to function, then nothing would ever be accomplished. Avoid letting your feelings control your function!

Your Health Status: How Did (Does) It Influence Your Performance?

- How is your general health?
- What is your frequency of illness?
- What is your frequency of common discomforts such as headaches or indigestion? (You can often control the intensity of these common discomforts if you act early—for example, at the onset of a headache—rather than later, when they reach an intensity at which you just can't think.)
- If you have a chronic health problem, do you put extra effort into actions for the prevention and the maintenance of your physical and mental functioning? Do you avoid people known to have the flu or a cold? Why expose yourself needlessly to jeopardize your utmost abilities for success?

Your Degree of Satisfaction with Your Preparation: How Did (Does) It Influence Your Test Results?

- Your attitude toward test preparation can make or break your performance on an exam. Be realistic and honest now and answer this question: Do you expect to know *all* of the content tested? Say no! And believe it! *All* is an absolute. Eliminate inappropriate absolutes from your value system by catching them in your day-to-day conversation. (For example, if someone says, "You always do that," counter with, "I'm not that perfect to do it *all* the time.")
- The bad news on exams, especially comprehensives, is that you will encounter items unfamiliar to you. Do you use tactics such as piloting your thinking and prioritizing to help you figure out the correct answer?
- Rather than negative statements about your preparation, use positive affirmations: "I've given my best, I'll go with what I know", or "I know some things, I'll figure the rest out."

What Can Your History of Testing Behaviors Teach You?

Keep a log or list, either mentally or in writing, of times of tension and fatigue during exams. Immediately after each exam ask yourself the following questions:

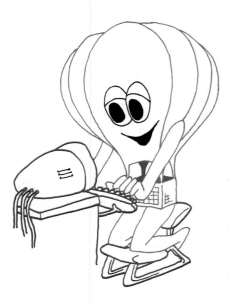

- During what part of the exam was I tense or tired?
- Did being tense or tired interfere with my thinking abilities?
- How did the number of questions affect the timing of my tension or fatigue?
- Did I have different reactions on the more specific versus the comprehensive or standardized exams? (See Chapter 11 for tips.)

Face the facts! Once you graduate, your exams will most likely be standardized. So prepare for these during your school days. From your log you will be able to map a pattern of tension and fatigue. Mapping your past patterns will provide clues for you to initiate changes during future exams. These changes, like the leather padding on the hot air balloon basket, will provide protection for a safe landing.

Repeat this inventory from time to time. Look at your history. What has your life in prior test situations been like? What about your life events before and after tests? Use this history of your behavior patterns to discern between those that work for you and those that work against you. See Chapter 5 for specific actions to deal with tension and fatigue.

HT Number Four: The How To's of Having Confidence

With confidence in old and new skills, what will be your new potential? Unlimited. The pilot knows when to turn on the heat for more hot air to increase the balloon's altitude. If too high, the pilot releases hot air through the specially designed deflation ports or vents and the balloon changes to a lower altitude.

In a like manner, you will need to adjust the heights of your confidence to maximize test performance: changing the *altitude* of your *attitude*. What do you say to yourself to boost your thoughts before, during, and after your test journey? How often do you inflate your mind with confidence-building behaviors and thoughts?

Are your confidence behaviors in moderation, neither over- nor under-inflated? Some people think you can't have too much confidence. But you can over-inflate your confidence without realizing that you might need to let out some air to approach a test situation more realistically. A "this is a breeze" attitude can set you up for frustration or a feeling of failure.

The worst tension and mind blocking sometimes occurs when a test is approached with the attitude of "I know *all* this content." Then, if the first five questions are about diseases you've not heard of, you panic. The remainder of the test becomes a blur, and your thinking freezes. You have not planned any alternative actions to bring yourself down and be able to "just read the question and select the best option." See Chapter 5 for specific actions to keep in reserve to combat this and other situations.

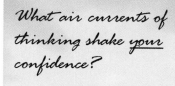

Avoid thinking like this: "I know or must know all the content."

On the other hand, is your fuel running low for some reason? Do you have minimal energy in reserve to boost your thoughts and behaviors in the confidence basket? Do you have a tendency to approach exams with an empty basket? (For example, "I know I didn't study enough. I never study enough or study the right things for tests.") Or do you get into different currents of thinking?

What air currents of thinking shake your confidence?

- The *"What if. . . ."*
- The *"I tried to study."*
- The *"I tried to do better."*
- The *"I tried not to change my answers."*

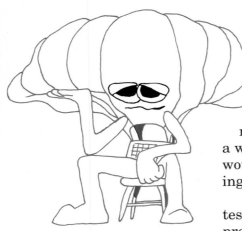

Either you do or you don't.

- The *"I tried not to get upset with stuff I didn't know."*

These statements with "try" in them are empty baskets of confidence! How would you like it if the pilot of your hot air balloon said "I'll try to fly this balloon," or a nurse said "I'll try to give you the proper shot," or a waitress said "I'll try to get your food for you." You wouldn't have much confidence in them. Even saying "I tried my best on the test" means nothing.

Successful test-takers either do their best on tests or don't do their best on tests. Be realistic. Be a producer. Eliminate the word "try." Counter those "try" types of thoughts with "I'll do my best!, I'll go with what I know!"; "I'm doing well, I'll keep on going!"; and "I've given my best during study times." Such positive affirmations become self-fulfilling prophecies.

Are you willing to take the risk? To learn from your mistakes and errors? To "do" instead of "try to do?" Consider this story of a test-taker:

"How did you get to be a successful test-taker?"
"Good judgment."

"How did you get good judgment?"
"Experience."

"How did you get experience?"
"Bad judgment." (Adapted from Aslett D, 1996)

A common question I get from students is: "I try not to change my answers on a test, but I keep doing it. How do I stop changing my answers?" I simply tell them this: *The best way to answer a question is to make a decision and go with it.* Learn to say the following as a habit, then carry it through to an action: "I will stick with my first answer. I will then go to the next question. I know I can change answers only when I can validate that I have truly misread the question, the options, or any given information." As you generate this new habit, talk about what you *will* do rather than what you *won't* do.

While doing practice questions, learn by not changing answers. Deal with the accompanying feelings (usually worry or tension) from this major change in habit. Some of you will have increased anxiety with this change in thought and behavior. However, with practice the anxiety decreases and eventually disappears. And you will find that you no longer fitfully change answers!

How do you gain confidence in test-taking skills? By learning to read and answer the questions precisely without the interference of over- or under-confidence. Keep doing questions at every opportunity: practice, practice, and practice. Do as few as five questions a day and use this four-step process:

1. Be a *detective.* Look for clues in the question, among the options, and in the information given. See Chapter 10 for more details.
2. Read *systematically.* Read the question first, then the options, then any remaining information in the stem.
3. *Read all of the options, then decide!* Sound simple? Maybe, but I'll bet you've missed a question or two from a knee-jerk reaction (read option *a,* know it's *the* answer, select it, and go on to the next question). Chances are that at one time or another you missed that question because option *d* was the correct answer. Remember to read *all* the options!
4. *Review practice questions.* Focus on the questions that you miss. Ask yourself the reason for your error in judgment. For example, "Did I miss the question from a lack of content knowledge? Or was there some other cause?" Most people fall in to the "other cause" category. See Appendix A to pinpoint your errors and perk up your test scores!

> Gain test-taking skills:
> - Be a detective.
> - Read systematically.
> - Read *all* options. Then decide.
> - Ask "Why did I miss it?" not "How many did I miss?"

HT Number Five—The How To's of Having Common Sense

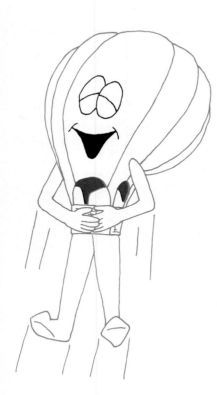

> *"A person without a sense of humor is like a wagon without springs—jolted by every pebble in the road."*
>
> *Henry Ward Beecher*

Common sense can be described as savvy, discernment, insight, or shrewdness. I think of common sense as ordinary logical thinking with an emphasis on the "thinking." You can sharpen your common sense in everyday life just by getting outside yourself and, depending on the situation, asking part or all of the following sequence of questions:

- What is the whole picture?
- What is the immediate situation?
- How does the immediate situation fit into the whole picture?
- What are other possibilities or actions?
- How might someone else see it?
- Is there a second right answer?
- Am I asking the wrong question?

Common sense skills are good to have. However, beware the trap of thinking to the point of "out-thinking" yourself or over-intellectualization. This can make you feel stuck or "grounded," unable to make a decision or act, with a feeling of paralysis. In other words, avoid overkill. Avoid letting over-analysis overwhelm your actions. Strike a balance between the situation and the time given for a decision. Keep it simple. It can be helpful at such moments to remember and practice this very simple sequence:

- See
- Think
- Act

Have a sense of humor. Laugh and learn from your errors. Avoid taking yourself too seriously. Lighten up! Remember this: it is the slack in the string that allows the kite or balloon to fly higher!

SUMMARY

Did you get a different view when you applied the Four Cs of test success to your familiar test prep landmarks? These Four Cs—content, control, confidence, and common sense—were discussed in order of priority and are similar to the four essential elements needed for a balloon trip—a balloon, maneuvering equipment, hot air, and the wind. Not one of them can be ignored. All four items are critical to success and incorporate the areas of physical, intellectual, and emotional preparation for tests.

The Five HTs—the how to's for content, control, confidence, and common sense development—provide specifics for improving test scores. Their intensity of growth provides a strong basis for your backup system when things go wrong (like mental blocks during tests). The challenge is for you to be dynamic in mind and body for test preparation and during tests.

"No farmer ever plowed a field by turning it over in his mind."
George E. Woodbury

Air Currents

"Some days we must function without feelings which might otherwise dictate our overall day or behaviors."

Dr. Paul Walker

"Life is like riding in an elevator. It has lots of ups and downs, and someone is always pushing your buttons. Sometimes you get the shaft, but what really bothers you are the jerks."

Roger von Oech

Piloting Your Thinking on Tests

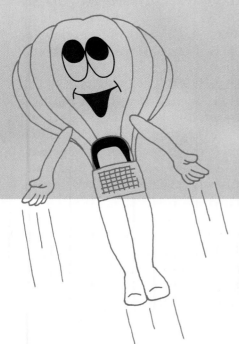

"You gain strength, courage, and confidence by every experience in which you really stop to look fear in the face. You must do the thing you think you cannot do."

Eleanor Roosevelt

What is *piloting your thinking?* In a nutshell, it is the disciplined process of actively and skillfully reorganizing your thoughts; it involves the following:

- Being focused on the test question at hand
- Avoiding thinking of the overall test
- Consciously leaving all other thoughts, whether of family, colleagues, school, or work, outside the exam room
- Leaving emotions or problems outside the door of the testing room

Note that all of these descriptions boil down to the same action: learning how to "shelve" all other thoughts except those that concern the issue at hand. This can be easier said than done. Sometimes, though, accomplishing this can be made more simple by imagining the act of actually setting these issues (often problems) down in a physical place. Be creative about this: Before a test, close your eyes and create an image of putting some problems on the floor of the exam room, leaving others in your car, on the back seat, the dashboard, in the trunk, or under the seat. Slowly "push" them farther back, or leave others on the counter at home.

The story is told of a man who worried about everything, even that he worried so much. He wanted to get rid of worry. So he developed for himself a Wednesday Worry Club to meet every Wednesday at 6 p.m. Whenever he found himself worrying about something, he wrote it down on a slip of paper and put in a box—the Wednesday Worry Club box. As he did so, he told himself he would not think of that issue again until the Wednesday Worry Club meeting. In this way, he put some of his worries out of his mind and into the box. When Wednesday came, he opened the box and read each worry. Surprisingly, he found that the majority of his worries had resolved themselves without his further efforts! (Peale, 1980)

What is the moral of the story? Before a test you must shelve, box, or wrap away any distracting thoughts or problems. Change your perception before tests by lightening your load of thoughts. Discard some thoughts; put others on the "back burner" of your mind to simmer in the unconscious and to be fired up about at a later, more appropriate time.

"Worry is an old man with bended head carrying a load of feathers he thinks is lead."

Corrie Ten Boom

ACTIVITIES TO PILOT YOUR THINKING

Once I learned to make use of this "back burner" or "shelving" process, I found it to be useful in many situations (for example, before I teach, in the middle of a day-long workshop, on my way home from work,

and before I do something that I enjoy). Try these activities to help you exercise this natural but often ignored skill:

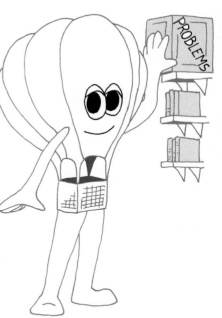

- *Make a picture in which you see yourself
  "shelving" your worries in a different way.*
  Picture them hanging in a tree on the school
  campus or out on a clothesline and strung out
  over a fence along the highway. Think of it as
  airing out your problems!
- *Do short bursts of work, during which you
  practice "shelving" or "shifting gears."* Work
  for 1 to 2 hours, then take a 30- to 60-
  minute break to do something you enjoy. During the breaks, shelve all thoughts of studying;
  while studying, shelve all other distracting
  thoughts.
- *Daydream or play.* When is the last time you
  really looked at the clouds just to watch how
  they move? What simple activities did you enjoy as a child? What activities, even now, can
  take you away into a daydream? As a child,
  what did you do to play? Get out some child-
  hood pictures to refresh your memory. Make a
  sign that reads: "Caution! Adult at play!"
- Playing, or having a little fun, produces energy
  for that next study session. (As you think of
  playing, are you tempted by TV? Evaluate
  whether television is really an effective break
  for you. Some people get caught up in channel
  surfing and never get back to work or study.)
- In any case, the next time you have a problem,
  play or daydream with it. If you don't have a
  problem, take time to play and daydream any-
  way. You may find some new ideas.
- *Stand, stretch, and channel surf your spec-
  trum.* Stand in a peaceful place (preferably
  outdoors), close your eyes (to rest them), do
  some deep breathing, and stretch. Your muscles get stiff just sitting and staring at a com-

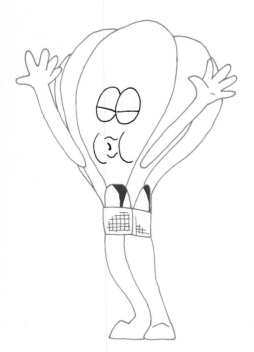

puter or textbook, even if you do tense/relax exercises and vary your eye focus every 15 to 20 minutes. You need to step away once in a while; stand and stretch your muscles.

- *Balance bad behaviors.* Be alert to those moments when you slide into the bad behaviors that lead to errors on tests. Substitute good behaviors that will be helpful to you during a test. Consciously use the nursing process as a framework for test preparation and during the test. Accept the behaviors you can change or maintain at this point in your lifetime. In other words, be realistic. Don't use behaviors you know will result in failure.
- When it comes to altering behaviors, think about selecting small things to do or think. Remember that the mighty oak tree came from a mighty small acorn! Recall that when a man is gloomy, everything seems to go wrong; when he is cheerful, everything seems right.
- *Listen to others.* Someone coming from a different viewpoint might offer ideas or advice on what to do, an action you never thought of, what *not* to do, or how *not* to do something.

HOW TO PILOT YOUR THINKING BEFORE AND DURING TESTS

Before a Test

Ask yourself the following questions:

- What is the purpose of the test?
- Is it a major or minor test?
- Is it specific or comprehensive?
- Does it count toward your grade?
- Does it determine if you pass, graduate, get licensed, or become certified?

If it is a *minor* test, expend minimal effort and time reviewing for it. Do plan to use both a physical and a mental exercise before, during, and after the test. Expect minimal tension and fatigue. (See Chapter 5 for these exercises.)

Plan for minor tests.

If it is a *major* test, give maximum attention to studying and reviewing. Begin preparation early by using a calendar. At the beginning of the quarter, mark the dates of all major tests. Use some type of symbol to designate study alerts. Make it a positive figure that is related to the content.

Plan for major tests.

Look ahead. Check your calendar each Sunday to preview the needs for that week and the remaining weeks in the quarter. Remember to limit your daily study time for each course. Stick to a 30-minute limit: this helps you to get to work and stay focused. Start with the most difficult content or course and finish with the easiest.

For a major test, plan to start studying at least 2 to 3 weeks in advance. Do some form of review for at least for 30 minutes on 6 days of the week (review your notes, read chapter summaries, review charts or pictures, or draw a picture of the physiology or pathophysiology). Don't forget to use 2 or 3 physical and mental exercises during study times. (See Chapter 5 for exercises.) Schedule 1 day off every week for yourself, for family or personal activities.

Expect to be easily distracted during study time for major tests. Many times, if we perceive a task as difficult, we have a tendency to put off working on it. Then, at the last minute, we try to cram everything in, ultimately crashing into fatigue and failure (not to mention feelings of guilt for not doing our best).

Expect maximum tension and fatigue up to a week before and during a major test. Delay any decision-making in other areas of your life at these times. Anticipate that your patience will be minimal, your common activities and common sense clouded. Don't be surprised if you wear one blue shoe with one

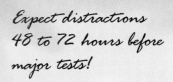

Expect distractions 48 to 72 hours before major tests!

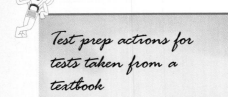

After tests, reward yourself with time or treats—no matter how you feel!

Test prep actions for tests taken from a textbook

green shoe, or lock your keys in the house. Remember not to take yourself too seriously at these times. Laugh at yourself and get the endorphins released rather than the epinephrine!

After the major test, reward yourself. Give yourself a gift of time or a small present. Take a couple of hours to just have fun and relax. I highly recommend a power nap of 20 to 30 minutes for the restoration of your mental and physical balance.

Know your instructor's testing style. If the instructor usually bases *75% or more* of the test questions on the book and less on the class notes, read the book first! Then review your notes and any other resources such as video or audiotapes. Reading the book before class may be the most helpful way for you to recall content. Try the express reading technique by reading your textbook in the following sequence:

- Introduction and objectives, if provided
- End of the chapter summary
- Major and minor headings throughout the chapter

As you do this, list on a note card the material that looks unfamiliar to you. Then go back and read in detail about this unfamiliar content. Read the familiar parts only if you have the time. If the instructor typically asks questions from the tables, charts, etc., now is the time to review these using the same sequence: major and minor headings, then the details of the content.

If the instructor usually bases *less than 25%* of the test questions on the book and most of the questions on class notes, read your book in the following manner:

- Introduction and objectives, if provided
- End of chapter summary
- Major and minor headings

Give more attention to your notes or audiotapes of the classes.

If it is a *comprehensive test,* such as the periodic achievement exams, use a different approach. Get a review text that has the content in an outline format along with questions and answers that include rationales for the correct and incorrect options. If you have time, schedule yourself to do the same number of test questions as on the comprehensive test (for example, 265 questions). Do the practice exam at the same time of day that the "real" exam will be. Use these practice comprehensive tests as a dry run for your licensing exam, even though it may be a few years away.

If your time before the test is limited, just do as many questions as you can within the time available for preparation. Keep a list on note cards of the material you missed. Use the test error work sheet presented in Figure 4-1 to help you track the material that you have trouble with. Whenever possible, use either the nursing process or the body systems as major headings. Most review texts will have the questions keyed as to the type of content.

Look up and review portions of missed content, organized by major headings, every couple of days rather than looking it up in bits and pieces on a daily basis. This technique, referred to as "chunking" material, results in better recall. Also, the outline format of the review book itself will help you remember the content better than other resources. If you need further clarification, look up the material in your textbook, not your class notes. If your class notes were taken on a bad day, they may be wrong or incomplete.

Be sure to get a good night's rest the night before comprehensive exams—at least 7 to 8 hours of sleep. These tests are usually longer and contain higher level questions that require more complex thinking.

If a test counts toward your grade, *know how much it is worth.* For a small amount of credit, such as 5% of a grade, it is probably not worth it to begin studying 3 weeks in advance. Instead, give more time for preparation to the bigger percentage tests.

Test prep actions for achievement tests

Know a test's worth— what percent of your grade is it?
The greater the percentage, the greater the amount of time required for preparation.

Test Error Work Sheet				
Question Missed	Did I not know the specific content? (Identify content)	Did I make a testing error in reading, comprehension, or perception?		
		Yes or no	If yes, was it in the question?	If yes, was it in the options?

Figure 4-1 Fill out the test error work sheet on a large index card to help you keep track of the material you have trouble with.

Balancing your review time this way helps you minimize or even eliminate tension and fatigue. You will have time to be your best on test day.

Have you ever felt very prepared for a test only to find that during the exam your mind froze and nothing could get it unstuck? Be prepared for this. Use mental and physical exercises, practicing them until they become second nature. Then during a test you can kick them into gear, make those difficult decisions, and do your best.

Does the exam determine whether you pass, graduate, get licensed, or become certified? Clear the area! Clear your calendar! This is serious business! As soon as you know the test date, mark it on your calendar and keep track of how many weeks there are to get ready. Then start planning to coordinate test preparation with other things going on in your life. Put these events on the calendar (include work days, days off, graduations, weddings, vacations—anything likely to take up a day or more of your time). The point is to be realistic about what other things are going on in your life before you write down a review prep schedule. If something seems to interfere and you can change it, do so. Delay any major decisions or activities, if possible.

Now look to see *realistically* what days on the calendar are left for test review and preparation. *Note that I said review, not study!* Comprehensive review is the better action for a comprehensive exam.

Next, as you prepare, remember that you can't know *everything!* If you don't know it by now, all the cramming won't help that "recall button" in your brain. It'll just put it out of commission. Approach test questions with the attitude, "If I don't know, I'll figure it out."

Make a separate review schedule for important comprehensive exams. Fifty percent of your prep time should be dedicated to the review of content. The other 50% should be for the practice of mental and physical exercises that focus on strategies to unlock

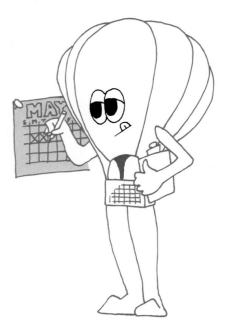

Clear your calendar for the big tests!

I can't and am not expected to know it all! When I don't know something, I'll figure it out!

mental blocks and physiological responses to test stress. Practice these strategies until you find that:

- They become second nature.
- You use a few exercises every day to cope with issues, stress, problems, or conflicts.
- Your rituals have positive results.

Exam Review Sessions: Two Samples

Two-hour Session

For a *2-hour* review session use the following steps:

Step 1. Sit for 5 minutes to empty your mind and re-lease tension from your body. Set a timer so you stay on track.

Step 2. Set the timer for 60 minutes. Do 60 questions. During this time do at least two sets of mental and physical exercises that take only 30 seconds (see Chapter 5). These exercises are recommended after the first 20 questions and then after question 40. *Answer each question and go on.* Do not leave questions to go back to others. If you get done early, take a break.

Step 3. Determine an average time per question (the number of seconds per question). Refer to Box 4-1, "Determination and Interpretation of the Time per Test Question."

Step 4. Take a 15-minute break before you correct the answers. Make sure you move around, stretch, and take a few slow, deep breaths as you stand and sit.

Step 5. Check your answers. At the same time, read the rationales for all of the questions—not just the questions you got wrong. Avoid correcting the entire test without reading the rationales. If you initially just correct the answers, you typically go on to calculate the percentage of correct answers. Calculations done at this point tend to distract your attention as you review the rationales! If the percentage of correct answers is high, you may tend to gloss over the rationales, thinking "I know this

Determination and Interpretation of the Time Per Test Question

1. Divide the number of test questions into the number of minutes it took you to complete the test. (For example, 60 questions divided into 40 minutes equals 0.66 of a minute per question.)
2. Multiply your answer by 60 seconds. (For example, 0.66 of a minute multiplied by 60 seconds equals 39.6 seconds for each question.)
3. What does this mean?

<25 Seconds Per Question

If you have an average time per question of less than 25 seconds, you are reading too fast! You are at risk of failing the test—not from a lack of knowledge, but from errors in reading, comprehension, or perception of what the question asks or the options state!

25 to 55 Seconds Per Question

You are within a time frame that promotes your abilities and knowledge for your best performance on any test.

>55 Seconds Per Question

If you have an average time per question of greater than 55 seconds, you are at risk of not completing the test. This time indicates that you either have a reading comprehension problem, that you have a tendency to read too much information into the question, or that you do not verify what the question is asking.

stuff!" If the percentage of correct answers is low, you may feel disgusted with your performance and have to review the rationales with increased tension, thinking "I'll never get this correct!" A reminder! Focus on the process, not the outcome at this time! Practice process thinking!

Step 6. Look at process issues for errors. After correction of the entire test, review each question that you missed. Make a test error list. This will pinpoint the decision-making errors that are detrimental to your goal of achieving higher test scores. See the work sheet on p. 56. Ask yourself the following questions about why you got the wrong answer:

- Did I not know the specific content?
- Did I make a testing error in reading, comprehension, or perception? Did I misread? If so, was it in the question or the options? What type of question or option was it? A priority question? An option with two parts?

Step 7. If you have time remaining in your 2-hour period, do more test questions, either one question at a time or in groups of five. At this time, plan to finish one question every 2 minutes. That gives you 1 minute to read the question and make a selection and 1 minute for the answer and rationale review.

Step 8. If you can, sleep for 1 to 2 hours after this 2-hour session so the material is centered into long-term memory (or take a 20 to 30 minute power nap).

All-day Session

For an *all-day* review, follow this schedule:

Step 1. Eat breakfast. Give yourself a leisurely 1 hour.

Step 2. Do a 2-hour review, following the schedule above.

Step 3. Take a nap or at least relax. Give yourself 2 hours off.

Step 4. Eat lunch. Give yourself a leisurely 1 hour.

Step 5. Do 2 hours of review, following the schedule above.

Step 6. Take a nap for 2 hours.

Step 7. Eat supper. Give yourself a leisurely 1 hour.

Step 8. Do 2 hours of review, following the schedule above.

Step 9. Go to bed for the night.

Step 10. Keep a list of missed content to identify a pattern of weak material. Do you have a knowledge deficit in any one step in the nursing process? In any one system of the body? In any communication or response phrase? In pharmacology?

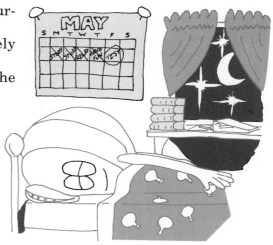

Critical Thinking and Test Exercise

You have probably heard about critical thinking. My guidelines and suggestions for test preparation and actions during test situations are grounded in the critical thinking process. Critical thinking basically means moving beyond simple memorization, knowledge recall, and comprehension into the areas of analysis, interpretation, and application of knowledge to real-life situations. As a process, critical thinking is dynamic and ever-changing, and results in further stimulation for a deeper understanding and a wider knowledge base of the subject matter. Using critical thinking to solve problems is similar to doing physical and mental exercises to control tension and fatigue (see Box 4-2). The more you use them, the more skilled you become.

Critical thinking means using _analytic_ and _interpretive_ skills, _applying_ knowledge to real situations.

> ### Box 4-2
>
> ### *Physical and Mental Exercises Immediately Before and During a Test*
>
> - Be quiet in mind and body.
> - Sit with your lower back against the back of a chair and place both feet flat on the floor.
> - Close your eyes.
> - Relax your hands. Have your hands in an open position and relaxed on a table or your thighs.
> - Breathe deeply and S-L-O-W-L-Y, in and out.
> - Consciously relax your muscles from head to toe with the expiration of your breaths. Lower your shoulders with each expiration.
> - Calm your mind and concentrate on the blankness inside your eyelids. Think about your mind's eye looking into a safe, peaceful emptiness. Think of a quiet scene—maybe at the beach or in the mountains.
> - Take one deep breath, tell yourself something positive, open your eyes, and return to the test question.

SUMMARY

Piloting your thinking involves "shelving" all distracting thoughts so that you can *focus* on the task, issue, or question at hand. *Before* an exam, this means planning or scheduling review sessions so that you can block out distracting personal issues, knowing that you have set aside time to devote to them later. This minimizes worry and physiological stress. *During* an exam, piloting your thinking involves using physical and mental exercises to help you really focus on the *immediate* question. As you practice answering exam questions, also focus on understanding answer rationales *(process thinking)* as opposed to merely calculating a score *(outcome thinking).*

Thinking: such a great asset to give you the edge for test preparation and test score improvement.

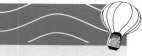

Air Currents

"Critical thinking further looks at these elements of thought which are implicit in all reasoning: purpose, problem/question at hand, assumptions, concepts, observed data (empirical grounding), reasoning leading to conclusions, implications/ consequences, objections from alternative viewpoints, and frame of reference."

R. Paul

"If you take too much time warming up, you'll miss the race. If you don't warm up at all, you may not finish the race."

Grant Heidrich

Detach Tension and Fatigue: Physical and Mental Exercises

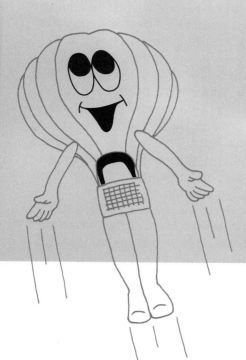

"Even as airplane engines must be tuned up before taking off, so must a human being have a tune-up process. The body has many miles of blood vessels and nerves to stimulate if you want to travel in high gear. And your mental and spiritual elements also require constant attunement to keep them functioning at full potential."

Norman Vincent Peale

Most students and graduates have varying degrees of tension or fatigue on a daily basis. A personal anti-stress regimen can be easily developed to minimize your stress response. Your focus for an anti-stress program should be to control how you react and respond to daily stressors, rather than on changing or

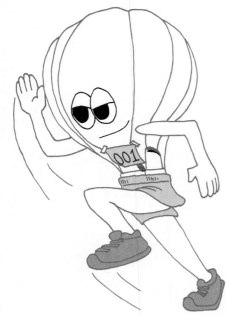

> *An anti-stress regimen decreases the effects of stress.*

> *Detach tension and fatigue—daily and weekly.*

eliminating the stressors. It is unrealistic to think that you can eliminate stress. However, you can either enhance or diminish the effects of stressors. Your anti-stress program should include the following key components:

- Convenience
- Time-effectiveness
- Inexpensiveness
- Fun

It should begin, of course, by including a well-planned program of diet, exercise, and relaxation.

When should you detach tension and fatigue? Do it on a daily and weekly basis. Then, during tests, your response to stressors will be automatic because you already routinely use the physical and mental exercises that you need in a test situation.

Remember how methodical you were when you first learned to drive a car? With practice, practice, and more practice, your thinking and reactions during driving became automatic in both normal and emergency situations. Similarly in test situations you will be able to control your tension and fatigue after practice, practice, and more practice of these physical and mental exercises.

When you achieve this level of control, you can maintain a minimum stress level so that your performance excels. You can answer test questions without cloudy or foggy mental activity. Performance in test situations excels when perceptions and decisions are accurate. You will be able to read the questions objectively, to think clearly, and to problem-solve. As with the initial nursing process step, you need to assess what influences your tension and fatigue during study, review of test questions, and during tests.

What are your stressors during tests? To be able to control your tension and fatigue, you must first identify what your stressors are during tests.

The three most common categories of exam stressors are:

- Mental
- Physical
- Psychosocial

What are *mental* stressors during tests? Mental stressors are those messages you play over and over in your mind. They are more commonly associated with content or knowledge issues. Frequently they may:

- Be of a negative nature
- Drain your confidence
- Drain your energy
- Interfere with your thinking ability

What do you do about mental stressors during tests? First, you have to consciously work at becoming aware of these messages. When you are aware of them, you can counter them with positive messages. But avoid thinking that you can eliminate all negative messages from your mind. We are humans, and this negative thinking is a human tendency. If you attempt to eliminate negative thoughts—an impossible task—the result may be an increase in mental and physical fatigue and tension.

Don't, for example, go in to take a test playing the mental message of "I didn't study enough. I know I'll have trouble on this test." Counter that thought with something more positive, such as, "I studied as much as I could. I know some content and will use that and critical thinking to figure out related items on the test."

Other positive messages might be:

- "I will slow down on the initial 15 questions and read the questions more carefully. I have butterflies in my stomach. Reading slowly initially will give me time to gather up the but-

Mental stressors are:
- *Replayed messages in the mind*
- *More often negatively focused*

"A man who removes a mountain begins by carrying away small stones."

Chinese proverb

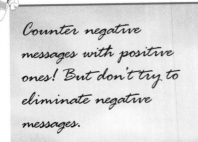

Counter negative messages with positive ones! But don't try to eliminate negative messages.

Physical stressors are:
* *The test environment*
* *Your bodily functions*

Psychosocial stressors are:
* *From interaction with others*
* *From those unwritten, invisible rules*

terflies in my stomach and get them to fly in the same direction."

* "I will ignore others in the room. If they leave early they've probably given up and didn't complete the exam."

What are *physical* stressors during tests? Physical stressors include both factors in the environment and your bodily functions. Take a few minutes to do the inventory and follow-up exercise for physical stressors presented in Figures 5-1 and 5-2.

What are *psychosocial* test stressors? Psychosocial test stressors may result from the behaviors or comments of your colleagues, financial obligations, family expectations, and employment needs.

Be alert to any detrimental comments from colleagues either during study or class time or right before the exam. Counter each of these comments with a positive one. You will be helping both yourself and your colleague.

Also, during an exam, be cautioned to avoid associating any friend's or family member's physical problems with your test material. Association of similar conditions may cause you to answer the question based on your personal experience rather than on fact or theory or on the information given to you in the stem of the question.

Family events, behaviors, comments, and interactions can raise issues of conflict before an exam. Your reactions to these conflicts may alter how you cope with or perceive questions on the exam. You may be so upset that you just can't think when it is time to take the test. It has nothing to do with preparation or knowledge. Being upset could result in an inability to perform, even at a minimal level.

Be prepared. Remember that you *cannot control* the behaviors of *others*. You cannot control your *reaction* to their behaviors. However, you can control your *response* to behaviors! You can put your reaction behind you and get on with the task at hand and give

Inventory of Physical Stressors During Tests

What are the characteristics of the exam room?

1. Temperature _____

2. Type of seat and desk _____

3. Noise level _____

4. Lighting _____

5. Type of test material (computer, paper and pencil) _____

6. Proximity to other test-takers _____

7. (Add your own) _____

What are your feelings and behaviors before and during tests?

1. Do you usually feel hot or cold?* _____

2. What foods do you eat before a test?** _____

   What foods have a negative effect on your bodily functions? _____

   How do they make you feel? _____

3. What beverages do you drink prior to a test?*** _____

   What beverages have a negative effect on your bodily functions? _____

   How do they make you feel? _____

4. Do you use any over-the-counter or prescription drugs? _____

   How do they make you feel? _____

5. (Add your own) _____

*I suggest that you wear layered clothing when you take a test. That way you can remove outer layers in case your body becomes too warm.
**Spicy, fatty, and high-sugar foods may result in sluggishness, heaviness, or indigestion.
***Caffeine may increase feelings of being "hyper," as well as tension and anxiety, and may also result in frequent trips to the rest room. Alcohol depresses the central nervous system and dehydrates and depletes the body of important minerals.

Figure 5-1   Use this inventory to determine the physical stressors that you must deal with during tests.

Follow-Up Physical Stress Exercise

Which physical stressors are in my control?

1. _____

2. _____

3. _____

Which physical stressors are uncontrollable?

1. _____

2. _____

3. _____

How could I control my response to the uncontrollable stressors?

1. _____

2. _____

3. _____

How could I prevent any of the physical stressors?

1. _____

2. _____

3. _____

Did any new actions to minimize physical stressors work for me?

_____

_____

What factors hindered my new actions and kept them from being effective?

_____

_____

Figure 5-2 Do this exercise after completion of the "Inventory for Physical Stressors During Tests." Ask yourself the above questions and list at least two answers at this time. You may want to return and add more later.

100% of your attention and efforts to the test preparation or situation.

> *Question:* After your self-assessment determines which test stressors you have, what do you do?
> *Answer:* Physical and mental exercises; they are the keys to unlocking your maximum potential.

A word of caution is needed here. Your goal is not to eliminate *all* anxiety. Everyone feels anxious before an important exam (which you may interpret as *all* exams). The feeling is normal. It can even be beneficial. A little tension or a little tiredness may be just enough to:

- Keep you alert
- Motivate you
- Help you to concentrate

Remember that the body systems and feedback loops rely on some degree of tension to function properly, much the way that the tension in a balloon's cables is necessary to carry the passenger basket. If the cables were cut, the basket would fall and the balloon itself would have no control because of the lack of *all* tension and stress. The old adage still holds true that "with the removal of all anxiety and stress, the result is a body that is dead." The goal is to keep your tension and fatigue harnessed and controllable.

If you have completed the Test Attitude Assessment in Chapter 1, keep your own needs in mind as you read through the physical and mental exercises presented in this chapter. Check those that you might like to practice.

- For those exercises that you already use routinely and find helpful, put a + in front them.
- Cross through those exercises that you've already tried and found useless.

What else can you do to control your reactions to stressors? Simply relax!

No stress = a person assuming room temperature. Think about it!

"It is as important to cultivate your silence as it is your word power."
William James

Here are some tips that work. Remember, however, that these need to be practiced on a daily basis so their effects can be the most useful to you at any time. (See Box 5-1 for a set of rules for the practice of physical and mental exercises.) Think of this time spent as investing your money in the bank of stress coping resources. Some of these exercises/actions can be done during a test as well as before a test. Prac-

---

Box 5-1

Rules for the Practice of Physical and Mental Exercises

- Do at least one physical and one mental exercise every day.
- Do both types of exercises at least three times a day: in the morning, in the middle of the day, and in the late evening before bed.
- Do exercises that take from 30 seconds to 30 minutes. Vary your exercises based on the available time. Anything over 30 minutes will most likely never be done on a consistent basis.
- Do them for at least 1 month before evaluating their effectiveness.
- Do a new exercise, either physical or mental, each month. Don't forget to keep doing the old exercises that work.
- Do a rotation of the effective exercises based on the situation, the availability of time or conditions, or just how you feel at the moment. For example, if it's raining outside and you have no umbrella, it may be foolish to decide on a 5-minute walk.
- Do at least one physical and one mental exercise before studying, doing any questions, or before a test in school. Select exercises that take only *60 to 90 seconds* in these situations so that you won't worry about using up too much time.

tice them all to see which ones fit into your daily schedule and bring results for you.

EXERCISES FOR TEST PREPARATION

Physical Exercises/Actions

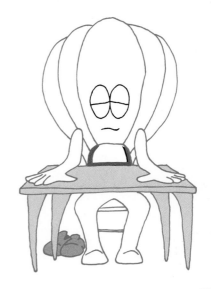

- **Eat** foods that help moderate your physiological stress. Vitamin C and citrus fruits help combat short-term intense stress. Protein, calcium, and potassium help offset the negative effects of long-term stress. Complex carbohydrates such as pasta, nuts, and yogurt can settle your nerves. Keep yourself in good health.
- **Relax** your hands. Close your eyes. Make a tight fist with both hands. Then put your hands into an open, relaxed position on top of a table or on the tops of your thighs.
- **Change** your footwear. Study in your bedroom slippers or favorite socks. Wear those favorite socks to the test. Or maybe, during the test, slip one or both shoes off while telling yourself to read the question as if you are in someone else's shoes.
- **Breathe** deeply and S-L-O-W-L-Y, in and out.
- Exercise your muscles. Work out stress through exercise. Engage in some type of exercise daily, even if it is just isometric exercises in the morning before you get out of bed. However, be careful with exercise and don't overdo it.
- **Exercise** your lungs. Do a breathing exercise. Close your eyes. Breathe normally through your nose. At the end of your exhalation, stop and count "one thousand one, one thousand two." While you count, focus on relaxing your body; let your shoulders slump and your hands fall open. Repeat the

Control during tests means:

- *Accurate perceptions and decisions*
- *Answering the test questions without foggy thinking*

Physical exercises stimulate your circulation as well as your brain for optimal thinking.

exercise until you have felt the tension leave and you are feeling relaxed.

- **Totally tense!** Sit in a chair in a darkened room. (If no dark room is available, just sit and close your eyes.) Start at your toes—curl them tightly. Move up to your calves—tighten them as tight as you can. Move up to your thighs—tighten them. Move to your buttocks—squeeze them together as tightly as possible. Remember to keep all the muscles tense as you go up in your body. Continue on to tighten your stomach muscles. Now move up to your arms—flex your arms with a tight fist made as the upper arms push inward into the chest wall. Move on up to your shoulders, which you now scrunch up, trying to touch them to your ears. Lastly, make the tightest face you are able. Don't forget to furrow your brow. Hold this position, totally tense from your toes to the top of your head, for 5 to 10 seconds. Then release all muscles quickly. You should feel a rush of blood into all of your muscles. This is a normal feeling. Repeat as needed to release any muscle tension or angry emotion from yourself. (Usually three times within 2 or 3 minutes is sufficient to get you physically relaxed and mentally refocused.) Once you have mastered this exercise, you can even do it in a standing position. Be careful, since this tension/relaxation of the muscles may result in a little dizziness from a slight transient drop in your blood pressure.
- **Slow down!** Just slow down in your actions. Become methodical. Act as if you are a robot.
- **Take** weekly extended relaxation. Do something with your family or friends at least once a week. Set aside this time as their time to do something together with you, even if it is only for 30 minutes. Create a balance between family, school, work, and relaxation.
- **Beware** of too much physical exercise. This can trigger the production of cortisol in your body,

which can cause an increased stress response. On the other hand, just the right amount of exercise can increase the amount of beta-endorphins in your system. These morphine-like chemicals produce a sense of well-being, reduce the sensation of physical pain, and counter the effects of negative stress hormones. The more you exercise, the longer these chemicals linger in your body.

- **Do** diaphragmatic breathing. Twice a day take 5 minutes to practice this type of breathing (do it before other exercises, if possible). Be aware that, commonly, your first practice sessions may leave you with a slight dizzy feeling for a few minutes. Don't strain to hold your breath or to go slower than is comfortable. In fact, at first you may prefer to do this exercise lying down. Good times to practice are before getting out of bed in the morning or as you go to bed at night. Later you may want to progress to sitting, then standing during this exercise.

The steps for diaphragmatic breathing are as follows:

1. Place one hand on your chest and one hand on your stomach or below your belly button.
2. Relax and breathe at a regular rate.
3. Feel which hand rises first when you breathe in.
4. Now, staying relaxed, breathe through your nose so that the hand on your stomach rises. To do this, you must breathe using your diaphragm. The hand on your chest may rise slightly or not at all.
5. Hold a second or two after inhaling fully; count "one thousand one, one thousand two."
6. Breathe out through your nose.
7. Repeat this exercise three to five times, then rest.

Pain, fatigue, tension, and poor movement habits may lead you to develop an abnormal breathing pattern called "shallow chest" breathing. In this type of breathing, the person usually has a forward head and shoulder posture and raises only the top of the rib cage to breathe. Breathing in this manner requires the small muscles in the neck to work excessively.

Mental Exercises/Actions

- Congratulate yourself daily on at least one of your accomplishments. For example, "I did five questions today and found time to relax for 10 minutes." Give one positive comment to each of your family members.
- Decide that you can interpret a situation in any way you choose. You don't have to rely on someone else's view.
- Imagine how you will look, feel, and act once you have accomplished little goals for the day or week.
- Accept things you cannot change. Pitch them out of your mind. Give them no time.
- Give negative thoughts, words, actions, and attitudes no time.

Combination Exercises/Actions: Both Physical and Mental Components

- Do a quiet exercise. Sit with your lower back resting against the back of a chair and place both feet on the floor. Close your eyes. Take a deep breath. Consciously relax your muscles from head to toe with the expiration of your breath. Lower your shoulders. Calm your mind and concentrate on the blankness inside your eyelids. Think about your mind's eye looking into a safe, peaceful emptiness.
- Take a mini-vacation in your mind. Close your eyes. Picture a pleasant, peaceful setting. Picture yourself in it. Concentrate on the happy or relaxed

feelings of your being in this setting (in your mind's eye). Then, take at least three deep breaths. As you breathe in, picture the word *calmness* going deep into your lungs' alveoli. As you breathe out, picture the word *tension* being vacuumed out from inside your lungs into the outside air. Repeat as needed. Before opening your eyes and returning to reality, turn off the picture of the pleasant setting. Have a blank screen on the inside of your eyelids. Focus on the nothing. Then open your eyes and return to the task at hand. With practice you can use this technique anywhere. Depending on your available time, this exercise can last from 15 seconds to 15 minutes.

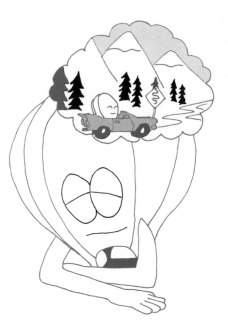

- Do a body scan with head-to-toe relaxation. Get into a comfortable position, either lying down or sitting. A good time to practice this exercise is just before you get out of bed in the morning or right after getting into bed at night. (This exercise works well for insomnia.)

  1. Close your eyes. The focus is to identify tense muscle groups then consciously relax them.
  2. Start at your forehead. Is it tense? Relax those frowning muscles.
  3. Go to your face next. Relax all of the muscles in it. Moving down let your head drop as you relax your neck muscles.
  4. Go now to the shoulders and hands. Are they tight or sore? Now have your shoulders slump as if a heavy raincoat is resting on them.
  5. Check out your upper extremities. Is there any tenseness there? Go ahead and relax your arms as if melting them into your thighs or into the table they rest on. Are you clenching a fist? Make your hands rest in an open position, as if you are catching money from the sky.
  6. Move to your abdomen. Now is the time to have a pooched-out, relaxed belly.
  7. Next go to your buttocks and thighs; picture them melting into the chair.

8. Finish up to see if your calves, ankles or toes are tense or sore. Make a conscious effort to have the muscles in them relax.

9. As you finish this head-to-toe relaxation, picture a trap door in the tip of each of your big toes. Have this trap door open and release all of the tension from your muscles.

10. Repeat the mental scan for tense muscle groups, again going from head to toe. Do this as many times as necessary until you feel relaxed or can fall asleep. With practice, these body scans can be done in 15 seconds to a few minutes for each part of the body.

11. Note the muscle group in which you find the greatest tension or the muscle group that is the most difficult to consciously relax. This is your particular area of the body where you store emotions of anger, sorrow, or irritation.

- Do nothing. Sit quietly. Think of nothing. If your eyes are open, concentrate on one small thing—maybe on the handle of a closet door or, if you're outside, on a blade of grass. As thoughts jump into your mind, push them out and continue to concentrate on the one small detail that you have chosen. Read Box 5-2 for suggestions.

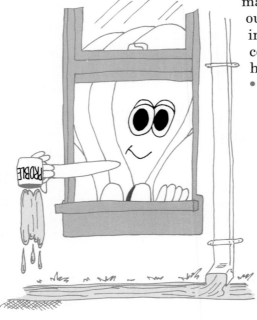

- Stuff the Cup and Dump! Pretend you have a cup in your hand. Now think of issues, situations, or people that have upset you. Recall that emotion. Now take that emotion and stuff it into the cup. Pack in as much as you can! Next, dump it into a garbage can, off the balcony, out of a window, or wherever is convenient to you at the time. Continue to stuff and dump! Keep doing these actions until you feel a sense of relief or a sense of being drained of that emotion. A variation of this exercise is to mentally stuff the issues, situations, or people themselves into the cup. Then dump them out! Some people

---

Box 5-2

The Practice of Silence

At some time during the day, it is a good thing to observe a period of absolute quietness, for there is a healing power in silence. Go to a quiet place. Do not do anything; throw the mind into neutral as far as possible; keep the body still; maintain complete silence. Beneath the tension-agitated surface of our minds is the profound peace of deeper mental levels. As the waves beneath the surface of the ocean are deep and quiet, no matter how stormy the surface, so the mind is peaceful in its depths. Silence has the power to penetrate to that inner center of mind and soul where God's healing quietness may actually be experienced.

Peale NV: *Stay alive all your life,* 1957. In Peale Center for Christian Living special edition, Pawling, N.Y., 1997, Simon and Schuster.

imagine taking their shoes off and grinding the negative emotions into the floor.

QUICK STRESS RELIEF EXERCISES DURING TESTS— 5 TO 60 SECONDS

The following breathing and stretching exercises can be done on a weekly or daily basis before tests, but they can also relieve tension or fatigue during a test.

- Breathing Variations
  1. Inhale for 4 seconds; breathe from the diaphragm.
  2. Hold for 20 seconds.
  3. Exhale for an 8-second count.
  4. Repeat three to five times.
  5. Practice four times daily.

- Head Turns
  1. As you sit in your chair, maintain good posture with your head erect and centered over your shoulders.
  2. Turn your head to one side as you keep your chin parallel with the floor; do not tilt your chin up or down.
  3. Breathe in and out as you hold this position for 5 seconds.
  4. Turn your head back to center and relax,
  5. Now turn to the other side; breathe in and out as you hold this position for 5 seconds.
  6. Turn your head back to center and relax.
  7. Repeat two to ten times on each side until you feel tension and fatigue decrease or disappear.
- Side Neck Bends
  1. As you sit in your chair, maintain good posture with your head erect and centered over your shoulders.
  2. Lean your head to one side so that your ear moves toward your shoulder.
  3. Keep your shoulders relaxed.
  4. Be sure to face straight ahead as you breathe in and out.
  5. Hold this position for 5 seconds.
  6. Return to the center position.
  7. Repeat exercise on the other side.
- Front and Back Neck Bends
  1. As you sit in your chair, maintain good posture with your head erect and centered over your shoulders.
  2. Lean your head forward until your chin comes close to or touches your chest.
  3. Keep your back straight.
  4. Breathe in and out while you hold this position for 5 seconds.
  5. Lift up your head to the center position and relax.
  6. Optional: lean your head backward.

7. Keep your back straight.
8. Breathe in and out while you hold this position for 5 seconds.
9. Lift up your head to the center position and relax.
10. Repeat two to ten times as needed until tension or fatigue is diminished.

- Side Chin Tilt
  1. As you sit in your chair, maintain good posture with your head erect and centered over your shoulders.
  2. Turn your head to one side as you keep your chin parallel with the floor.
  3. Lift your chin as tolerance allows, as though you were looking up toward the ceiling.
  4. Breathe in and out as you hold this position for 5 seconds.
  5. Lower your chin, then turn your head back to center and relax.
  6. Now turn to the other side and repeat maneuver as above. Breathe in and out as you hold this position for 5 seconds.
  7. Turn your head back to center and relax.
  8. Repeat from two to ten times on each side until you feel your tension and fatigue decrease or disappear.

- Shoulder Rolls
  1. Sit with your arms at your sides.
  2. Breathe as you raise your shoulders up and forward.
  3. Continue this shoulder motion to roll them toward your ears.
  4. Hold for a moment.
  5. Breathe out as you roll your shoulders backwards and down to the starting position.
  6. Relax for two or three deep breaths; then repeat this exercise two to ten times or until you feel your tension and fatigue decrease or disappear.

- Shoulder Rotations
  1. Sit in a chair that provides good support.
  2. While keeping your elbows at your sides and at a 90-degree angle, rotate your arms outward.
  3. You should feel your shoulder blades squeeze together.
  4. Hold for up to 5 seconds, as tolerated.
  5. Repeat as needed. This exercise may also be done in a standing position.
- Tense-Relax Exercises
  1. Do three to five abdominal breaths.
  2. Sit with your lower back against the chair and both feet on the floor.
  3. Clench your fists.
  4. While continuing the fist clench, pull your forearms tightly up against your upper arms.
  5. Keeping those muscles tense, tense all the muscles in your legs as well.
  6. Keeping all of these muscles tense, tighten the muscles in your face and shut your eyes (but not too tightly).
  7. Now, while continuing to tense all these muscles, take a deep breath and hold it for a count of five.
  8. Now let everything go all at once! Let the muscles go. Let them totally relax. Feel yourself letting go of all of your mental tensions as well as the physical tensions. Enjoy the feeling of relaxation for a minute or two.
  9. Repeat this exercise two or more times consecutively during a test if you feel yourself becoming tense or tired.
- Chin Tucks
  1. As you sit in a chair, maintain good posture with your head erect and centered over your shoulders.
  2. Actively tuck your chin in.
  3. Pull your head backward while continuing to face forward.
  4. Do not tip head up or down.

Box 5-3

Guidelines for Sitting at a Computer Desk

1. Ask for a chair with arm rests.
2. Adjust the chair height to avoid stress on your wrists, forearms, and neck. (Ideally, your arms should be near your sides and your elbows at a 90-degree angle.)
3. Adjust the chair or computer screen so that the screen is at eye level so your neck is not constantly bent. (Don't forget to do your eye exercises frequently.)
4. Ask if a stool is available to rest your feet on, especially if it seems you will be there for the duration of a 5-hour licensure examination.

---

5. Hold for a count of five as you breathe in and out.
6. Return to the neutral position and relax.
7. Repeat 15 to 25 times.
8. Doing this in the shower helps to loosen those tight neck muscles.
9. Do this three times a day in preparation for computer exams (see Box 5-3 for other computer test-taking tips).

SUMMARY

You can easily develop a personal anti-stress regimen to minimize your stress response. Remember, stressors are present every day. Whereas you have no control over *them,* you do have control over how you *respond* to the stressors. You can either enhance or diminish the effects of stressors. "Daily detach your tension and fatigue." Key components of your anti-stress program should be convenient, time-effective, inexpensive, and fun. The best plan should also include careful planning for a balanced diet, as well as exercise and sufficient relaxation.

Finally, the 30- to 60-second exercises or actions that work well during tests—especially during computer testing—are the following:

- S-L-O-W deep breathing at least three times at any given instance.
- Closing your eyes and thinking of nothing for 5 to 10 seconds.
- Taking a mini-vacation in your mind.
- Just slowing down.
- Totally tensing then relaxing.
- Doing a head-to-toe body scan.
- Taking your shoes off (while thinking of being in someone else's shoes).

Air Currents

"The food that enters the mind must be watched as closely as the food that enters the body."

George E. Woodbury

"Pleasant sights give health and happiness."

The Way

"Internal balance is health and internal imbalance is sickness. These bodily functions are controlled by glands that are influenced by mental health."

Dr. Clarence Cook Little

6

The Position, Priorities, and Killer Questions

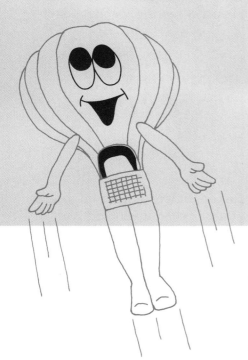

"When those 'killer' questions get you down, it's time to lighten up. Ease up and don't push too hard. Don't dwell on the past, missed 'killer' content. Look forward. Have a sense of humor and keep your heart at peace."

Adapted from Norman Vincent Peale

WHAT IS "THE POSITION"?

Get Into "The Position"

When *priority-setting* in studying and in doing practice questions, it is essential to think of your physical and mental preparation for a test. This preparation can be facilitated by "the position." Studying, just like a sports activity or a hot air balloon trip, requires that you get into "the position" before taking action.

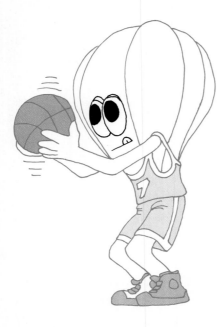

- Think about a baseball player who swings the bat a few times before getting into "the position" to hit the ball.
- Think of a basketball player who dribbles the ball a few times before getting into "the position" to take a foul shot.
- Think of the balloon being stretched on the ground, then checked for rips and tears, then the basket being carefully connected to the balloon ("the position") before launch.

It is essential that you develop "the position" for yourself before you begin to study or to take a test. This position is also effective in combating tension or fatigue during study, review, testing, or just listening to a lecture.

WHAT ARE THE PRIORITIES FOR YOUR DEVELOPMENT OF "THE POSITION"?

Get On Your Mark!

Let's explore a little further the position that would get you off to a jump start. I recommend that you sit in a comfortable chair or on a sofa.

- Both of your feet should touch the floor.
- Your lower back and hips should rest against the chair or sofa.
- No crossing of the legs at the ankles or knees is allowed initially.
- Your arms should be relaxed and rest on your thighs or on a table in front of you.
- Your hands should be in an open position without any degree of clenching your fist.

This is called the "Get On Your Mark!" position.

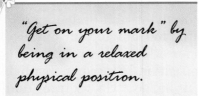

Get ready to study and take tests by getting into "the position." It is the signal to "get focused."

"Get on your mark" by being in a relaxed physical position.

Get Ready!

Once in the correct, relaxed physical position, the next step is to double-check for tension.

- Close your eyes.
- Think of nothing.
- Push all thoughts out of your mind.
- Concentrate on the blank space inside of your eyelids.
- Now do a head-to-toe scan for any tense muscles or any awkward positioning of your extremities.
- If any tension is found, make a conscious effort to relax that muscle group.

This is called the "Get Ready!" position.

"Get ready" by checking yourself for residual mental and physical tension.

Get Set!

After you have verified that you are completely mentally and physically relaxed and not thinking of anything, do one last set of actions before opening your eyes.

- Take three S-L-O-W, methodical, deep breaths.
- As the air goes into your respiratory tract, picture the parts of the respiratory tract and even feel it as the air is inhaled and exhaled.
- At the end of exhalation, count "one thousand one, one thousand two," then progress into the next S-L-O-W, deep breath.
- On the third inhalation and exhalation, mentally say to yourself one positive statement about the study or test event. Examples are: "I only have 20 minutes to study; it will be the best 20 minutes I've ever done." "I know some material. On the questions I don't know, I'll figure it out!"

"Get set" by flushing the negatives from your mind with enthusiasm and optimism.

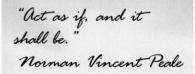

"Act as if, and it shall be."
Norman Vincent Peale

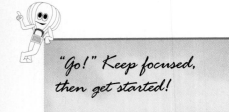

"Go!" Keep focused, then get started!

- Say these to yourself with enthusiasm and conviction.

This is called the "Get Set!" position.

Go!

You know what follows now. Open your eyes and "Go" to studying or taking a test! To recap, recall the actions that go with these positions:

1. Get on Your Mark!
2. Get Ready!
3. Get Set!
4. Go!

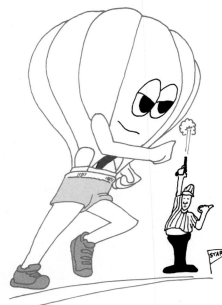

You should do this sequence of actions before every study session or test. Doing them will help you focus on the task at hand. Compare yourself to successful athletes, individuals who readily talk about their need to be focused to do their best. Get focused, then get started!

WHAT ARE THE PRIORITIES WHEN YOU STUDY?

Priority-setting is as essential for test preparation as for the first balloon flight. Test preparation begins with priorities based in three areas: intellectual, physical, and emotional. Intellectual endeavors should be done first. Nothing beats the three basic rules that start with "sit down." They are as follows:

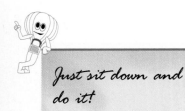

Just sit down and do it!

1. Sit down and review before a test.
2. Sit down and do practice test questions.
3. Sit down and learn from your mistakes.

Now consider the physical and emotional aspects of test preparation. There is a way to prioritize what and how you study.

HOW CAN YOU USE PRIORITY-SETTING FOR STUDYING?

First, identify what tested material you feel comfortable with. If you are studying for a unit test, review the major headings in the chapters covered on the test. If reviewing for a comprehensive test, look over the table of contents of your text or review book. Use the following simple steps:

Prioritize your studies by dividing material into "need to know" stuff and "I know this" stuff.

1. Place a check mark in front of those headings you feel good about—the "I know this" stuff.
2. Place a circle in front of those headings you just can't remember—the "need to know" stuff.
   - Prioritize this material:
     Place a 1 in front of the heading that you think you need to study first.
     Place a 2 in front of the next heading and so forth.
3. On the material you think you know, there is no need to prioritize the major headings. However, I suggest that you find some time later to review the easier material. I have found these two approaches most effective:
   - Head-to-toe approach for body systems
   - Alphabetical approach to the organ systems

These approaches may need to be varied depending on the material being studied. For pediatric and maternity nursing, it is usually most efficient to use a chronological structure or a time-line associated with developmental criteria.

On high-energy days select the most difficult content to study or review. On low-energy days select the easier content to study or review.

WHEN SHOULD YOU STUDY/ REVIEW THE DIFFERENT CATEGORIES (OR PRIORITIES) OF MATERIAL?

The "Need to Know" Stuff

To be most efficient and effective, study/review the "need to know" material on high-energy days. These are the days when you feel great and think that you can do anything. Incorporate at least 1 to 2 hours of review time at one sitting on these days. Don't forget to do your physical and mental relaxation exercises before, during, and after the review period. The exercises will make your efforts even more effective.

The "I Know This" Stuff

Do the "I know this" stuff on your low-energy days (when you feel that nothing is going well and little energy is left in your body). Limit the study time to 15- or 30-minute increments. Perhaps take a 45-minute nap between study times, if time is available. On these days you need to incorporate your fatigue-busting exercises at least every 1 to 2 hours throughout the day.

What about those times when energy is at a moderate level and you find yourself wondering "What to do?"

- Do I review my notes?
- Read my text?
- Listen to my audiotapes from class?
- Do practice questions of the material to be tested?

The answer?

- Do test questions!
- Do test questions!
- Do test questions!

Doing test questions is the best exercise for your cerebral muscles.

Let the questions you miss be your guide, whether to go reread your notes or to look up the answers in your text. During this time you can also identify your pattern of test-taking errors. Thus at any given time you are working on two aspects of testing: content review and test-taking skills.

HOW CAN YOU USE PRIORITY-SETTING TO ANSWER "KILLER" TEST QUESTIONS?

Two schemes can guide your decision on the best option: (1) the format of the question and (2) the search for essential concepts.

Caution! These will not be used all the time or on every question. Use your common sense, logical thinking, and what you know to decide on a scheme.

Set priorities by focusing on:
- *The question format*
- *Essential concepts*

WHAT IS MEANT BY THE FORMAT OF THE QUESTION? HOW DO ESSENTIAL CONCEPTS FIT IN?

There are two types of question formats that result in "killer" or difficult types of questions. Both of these formats require you to determine whether all or some of the options are correct and just what the question is asking. And, as we shall see, interpretation of both types can be aided by clues in the form of these essential concepts:

Type 1 Question Format

These are questions that ask for:

- Initial or first action

Narrow the options to two. Then look for clues regarding:
- *Time elements*
- *Developmental sequences*
- *Acute versus chronic disease*
- *Related essential concepts*

- Priority factors or actions
- Identification of initial or beginning symptoms or signs
- Anticipated findings

These questions require you to consider all of the options as correct. Typically, all of the options will be correct answers. To read type 1 questions with the intent to find an incorrect option is an error in reading.

These are considered to be the harder questions because most test-takers can easily narrow the options to two. Once this is done, the test-taker should consider these additional priorities:

- Is there a time element?
- Is there a sequence of human development?
- What is the length of the disease process (acute or chronic)?
- What are the associated essential concepts? Although there are others, the essential concepts most frequently used are these:
  1. Maslow's hierarchy of needs (physiologic needs take priority over safety and love/belonging needs)
  2. Kübler-Ross' death/dying or loss theory (a process of denial, anger, bargaining, depression, and acceptance)
  3. The ABCS of airway, breathing, circulation, and safety.
  4. Internal versus external factors
  5. Acute versus chronic versus terminal

Type 2 Question Format

Another problem format is the awkwardly worded question. These types of questions challenge the reader to clarify just what is being asked. Some examples of awkwardly worded questions are the following:

- "What does the nurse include about what to avoid?"
- "The nurse would assess for all but which of these findings?"

The best approach is to first accept that there may be a few of these questions on the exam. Then decide to *avoid getting upset* over them. If you do get rattled, simply do a physical and mental exercise to get yourself refocused.

When you are focused, reword the question after first reading the options. Look for the sentence construction of subject, verb, and object. The above questions can be reworded to:

- "What should the client avoid?"
- "What would the nurse *not* look for?"

Now, do the following question and options for practice:

> If a nurse is in the process of ambulating a client, the nurse should discontinue the activity for all but which of these findings?
> a. Any drop in heart rate or blood pressure
> b. Any increase in heart rate or blood pressure
> c. A change of skin color to pallor
> d. A change of skin color to rubor

One rewording of the above question might be: "With which finding would the nurse decide to continue the activity?" Another approach is to use a two-step process to answer the question:

1. Reword the question to an opposite meaning: "What would cause the nurse to discontinue the activity?"
2. Then select three of the options to answer the reworded question. The option that is left is the correct answer.

Another essential concept that may apply to this sample question is the ABCS (of airway, breathing, circulation, and safety).

Avoid getting upset over convoluted test questions.

Try rewording difficult questions.

Search for essential concepts like the ABCS:
- *Airway*
- *Breathing*
- *Circulation*
- *Safety*

This particular question illustrates the use of the ABCS scheme. In the question and in the options, breathing and circulation changes take priority. Safety is of no concern in this question. Eliminate options *a* and *b*, which are associated with circulation and are each a priority. With these types of findings, the activity would be discontinued. Of the remaining options, you now have to decide on one of two colors—pallor or rubor.

If you have no idea of the correct answer, go with what you know, plus common sense. If skin has pallor, it reflects constriction of the blood vessels. You know this from your studies and possibly from the personal experience of being cold.

Perhaps you don't know what rubor is. Again, go with what you know. Based on what you associated with pallor—vessel constriction—this means blood is not getting to the tissues. This is reason enough to stop the activity, so eliminate option *c*.

So select the only option left, option *d*. Rubor means a ruddy or red color. If your skin is red, the vessels are dilated and blood is getting to the tissues. Of the given options, this is the least dangerous to the client.

HOW CAN YOU USE THE NURSING PROCESS TO STUDY/REVIEW OR DO TEST QUESTIONS?

The Nursing Process Applied to the Studying Process

In this chapter and others the nursing process is used to guide you in your study and test preparation activities. Here's how to apply it:

Assessment

You are encouraged to assess your preferences for:

- Test material
- Behaviors
- Thoughts about studying, reviewing, and testing

Use this assessment to identify the internal and external factors that influence your ability to perform under the pressure of testing. Increase your awareness of when and why you experienced fatigue or tension during exams.

Analysis/Planning

Decide what mental and physical actions work best for you and in what situations. Plan a daily schedule of study, doing practice test questions, and spending time for yourself and your family.

Intervention

In Chapter 5, it was suggested that various actions and exercises be performed daily for a month.

Evaluation

You are advised to evaluate the effectiveness of any changes you made in studying, doing test questions, and spending some time for fun things. Ask yourself, "What has proved to be the most effective for me?"

Apply the nursing process to study, review, and test questions:
- *Assessment*
- *Analysis/Planning*
- *Intervention*
- *Evaluation*

The Nursing Process Applied to Test Questions

With some test questions, the steps in the nursing process can direct you to the correct option. If the options contain various steps of the nursing process, the option that has an assessment behavior is probably the correct answer. Assessment is the first step for further action in nonspecific situations.

However, if comprehensive assessment data is given in the stem of the question, then the correct option is likely to be an analysis/planning or an intervention option. If you find yourself in doubt on a test question, "to do further assessment" is likely the best answer. Do the following question:

A child has swallowed an alkali solution. The goal for the nurse is to:

a. Neutralize the substance
b. Identify the specific solution
c. Prevent scarring/obstruction
d. Provide emotional support

Which option did you select? Many students have a knee-jerk reaction after reading the question and *option*. I say *option* because the first option appears to be correct. Did you fall into the trap? Did you select option *a* because it sounded correct? How closely did you read the question?

Remember to use the nursing process: Collect *all* assessments! Not just the ones you anticipate or want to hear.

Now, reread the question and all of the options.

Did you see the key word "goal" in the question? Option *a* is an intervention! Yes, you are correct in thinking of it as an intervention to prevent scarring, which could lead to obstruction. However, the correct answer for this question is option *c*, which is the goal.

The other options may be appropriate. However, the ABCS theme for priority-setting could be applied here. It is important to maintain a patent airway before identification of the specific substance or emotional support. (Remember Maslow's hierarchy? That could apply here, too.)

SUMMARY

In summary, stick to the basics. "Get on your mark"—what you need to review first when you sit down. "Get ready"—both physical and mental exercises. "Get set"—a last chance to clear your mind and do your best. Remember that "haste can make waste" no matter how much preparation has been done. Then "Go"—get focused. Simply read the question! Read the options. Narrow to two options. Use priority-setting and the ABCS approach. Make a decision. Go forward and never think back or look back to prior test questions!

Air Currents

Optimism: A cheerful frame of mind that enables the teakettle to sing a song even though it is in hot water up to its nose.

Author unknown

"Find out before you start beating something to death how dead it has to be, and work until you're there and move on."

D. Aslett

Tethering Lines for Remembering What You Want to Know

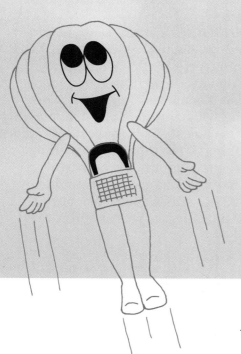

"Once upon a time, two frogs fell into a bucket of cream. The first, seeing that there was no way to get any footing in the white fluid, accepted his fate and drowned. The second frog didn't like that approach. He started thrashing around in the cream and doing whatever he could to stay afloat. After a while, his churning turned the cream into butter, and he was able to hop out."

Roger von Oech

What is the moral of the story above?
Be persistent! How persistent are you?

"Nothing in this world can take the place of persistence. Talent will not; nothing is more common than unsuccessful men with talent. Genius will not; unrewarded genius is almost a proverb. Education will not; the world is full of educated derelicts. Persistence and determination alone are omnipotent."

Calvin Coolidge

Part of being a good balloon pilot is developing strategies for harnessing that unpredictable natural force that is both its most helpful element *and* its greatest threat: the wind. Harnessed for use by the pilot, the wind not only becomes the key to speed and direction but also helps pilots set world records now and then. Out of control, the wind can cause devastation (shut down a flight or, at a minimum, impede success).

The same dilemma applies to the memory. Harnessed for use by the test-taker, the memory becomes the key to speed and direction in problem solving, and can even help the test-taker break his or her personal record on test scores. Out of control, the memory can become blocked and simply shut down. Both pilot and test-taker must develop a repertoire of strategies for harnessing and accessing their most important natural forces.

You can study. Or you can study and remember. Simple behaviors can make the difference. Different strategies are nice to know and helpful in handling the variety of material you need to remember. This chapter discusses several types of study strategies in addition to offering general guidelines. After establishing some key study tips, we'll look at strategies for note-taking, audiotaping, storytelling, imagery, and associations, and, finally, how to overcome mental blocks through the use of brain dominance. But first, Box 7-1 offers some last minute study tips for those times when you are in a real crunch.

STUDY SESSION TIPS

Before moving on to more specific memory-enhancing tools, it is appropriate to establish some overall study tips and behaviors that are helpful to adopt.

Box 7-1

Last-Minute Study Tips

- On the day before the test be sure to read over your class notes one last time to identify any gaps in material and specific instructor notes of what you "must" know.
- Study before sleeping, since this tends to set the information into long-term memory.
- Use commercially available review cards. Highlight hard-to-remember material in yellow or lime green and carry the cards with you so that you can fit in short study sessions at times of unexpected waiting.
- Put the review cards on the sun visor in your car. Reading over a few cards is a great time passer when traffic is at a stand still. Keep a few blank index cards with these, along with a pen to jot down content that needs further reading, review, or reinforcement.
- Color is important for the retention and recall of content. Use highlighters that are in the colors of yellow or lime green. Research on how colors affect memory and recall suggests that these are more effective to get the job done. Use a note pad with yellow pages instead of white. Use yellow note cards or sticky notes. Put them in places you frequently pass to remind you of material you want and need to know.
- Review in your text the end-of-chapter summaries and the major and minor headings.

Don't Forget to Move!

After every hour of study you must get up and move! Take a 5- to 10-minute break. This is especially important during an all-day study marathon. Of course,

Movement of the body massages the mind. Move! Study! Move!

all-day study is not recommended. But if you have to do it, follow these guidelines:

1. If you just can't get up and move, then set the timer and take a nap on your break time.
2. If you can, force yourself to do some type of physical activity every hour.

Don't think about anything; just do something physical. It's amazing how inviting chores begin to look when you are studying! It's even more marvelous to realize how much you can get done in such little time. Try one or more of these on a break:

- Put a load of clothes in the washer or dryer.
- Sweep the kitchen floor.
- Clean off the table or counter tops in the kitchen.
- Write out a few checks to pay the bills.
- Walk around the room.
- Look at a picture or accessory while you think of the happy memories associated with it.
- As you walk from room to room in your home, stretch your arms to the ceiling, then hug yourself, then stop and bend over to let your arms hang down and swing from side to side like an elephant's trunk.
- Look out the window with the intention of seeing something new or different (a bird, a squirrel, a flag, or changes in the color of the sky, in the leaves on the trees, or in the patterns of the clouds).
- Move to a different room. Sit and listen to some uplifting music. (Pick the type of music that gives you some energy!) As you listen, do deep breathing or move to the beat of the music. Concentrate only on the pleasurable sound of the music, or the air moving up and down your airway and in and out of your lungs.

Stretch your body's muscles as well as your mental muscles to prevent clots and constipated thoughts.

- Make a conscious effort to relax all muscle groups.
- Let your shoulders slump as if you have on a heavy raincoat.
- Move to the music. Dance. Or simply stand and bend your knees to the beat. Just keep moving!

Stop and Stretch!

Every 15 minutes during study periods, stop and stretch. Count to 10 as you perform each of these motions:

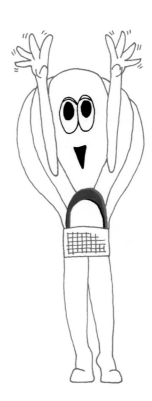

- Arms up to the ceiling with hands open and fingers moving.
- Arms down and shoulders pulled up as if trying to touch your ears with your shoulders.
- Shoulders down; now tighten the buttocks.
- Relax the buttocks and now dorsi flex one foot while you plantar flex the other foot. (This takes concentration and coordination! If you can't do the opposites, do both feet together. This exercise will help prevent clot formation in your lower legs.)

Recall question: Did you forget what direction the foot travels in dorsi or plantar flexion?

Recall tip: For dorsi flexion, think of the dorsal fin of a fish—it stands up out of the water. Think of a shark, and how most people first recognize them by the dorsal fin sticking up in the water. Dorsal fin is up—foot travels up. If you can remember this, just tell yourself that plantar flexion is the opposite.

For plantar flexion, if you can't remember the one above, think of planting a flower into the ground and tamping the soil down with your foot. The direction of the ground is down. Thus plantar flexion is down—the motion to plant the flower down into the ground.

Use Consistency in Study Sessions

Establish a consistent time every day to study, and study in the same place. If this can't be done every day, then shoot for three times a week. Consistency of time and place helps to keep your mind focused.

Dealing With Fatigue: Don't Fight It, Fix It!

Don't fight fatigue. Fix it!

If you cannot avoid the causes of your fatigue, you can still choose to alter your internal state. Score your fatigue on a scale of 0 to 10, with 0 equal to no fatigue and 10 equal to overwhelming fatigue. Calculate your level before and after each strategy.

Next, try some directional thinking. Say, "I can do something now to renew my energy"; or, "What enlivens me?"; or, "I am relaxed!"; or, "All my fatigue is leaving with my expirations!" Talk to yourself with enthusiasm!

Relax your muscles. In your mind, give yourself the world's best back rub or neck rub. Imagine all the right places being massaged perfectly.

The Quiet Place

Go to a quiet place where you can be alone and think, whether it's outdoors under a tree or in the shower. Close your eyes and relax your muscles as you take a few slow, deep breaths.

When you feel yourself completely relaxed, make positive, believable suggestions to yourself such as the following: "When I get back to studying, I will feel a new sense of energy and be focused"; or, "As I return to studying, a calm will encircle me. I will be able to think, be more alert, be refreshed."

Stick to statement possibilities that keep you in control. It is surprising how effective such suggestions, made to yourself when you're relaxed, can be.

If you should slip into self-discussions about "feeling tired," dispute them. Say, "This feeling, too, shall pass, as it has before" (Grainger, 1990).

The Energy Position

Assume a "position of energy" during study time: head up, shoulders relaxed, spine straight.

Take visual breaks every 3 to 5 minutes, or more frequently if your work is intense (for example, reading, working at a computer terminal, or writing notes).

Preventing Eye Fatigue

Make it a point to blink and take deep breaths. Sometimes intense work can prevent you from proper breathing and regular blinking.

If you plan to work with questions or content on a video display terminal, plan to vary your tasks to eliminate long periods of more than 1 to 2 hours at the terminal. If you wear glasses and are sensitive to glare or flicker, tinted lenses can help. Some people find that the kind of polarizing filters that mount on the screen are helpful in minimizing eyestrain.

Consider using a terminal screen with a light background and dark characters.

A yellow background with black letters works very well.

Take "look away" breaks. Change the eyes' focus by looking away into the distance. This relaxes the pupils.

Review question: If the pupils are relaxed, are they dilated or constricted?

Recall tip: Think of yourself when you are relaxed on the sofa or bed. Is your body position open and slung over the sofa, or is it in a tight, fetal-type position? Most people relax by spreading out on the sofa or

Quiet places recharge batteries in both the brain and the body.

Energy is emitted when you are in an upright position.

bed. The pupil takes a similar position with relaxation; it dilates and takes up more space in the eye.

A working, stressed pupil becomes small, pinpoint, or constricted. This is why intense, prolonged, close-up work results in headaches if "look away" breaks are not taken.

Home, Sweet Home

Change your environment at home. If you fall into your favorite chair as soon as you walk through the door, place your notes or a textbook on that chair in the morning before you leave. On your return you will have to move these things to sit down. Hold onto them and flip through them as you are flopped down in the chair.

Tell yourself to give the textbook just 5 minutes of your time. Before you know it, 15 or more minutes will have passed and you have successfully fooled yourself; the "get home flop" has become a "functional, fun flop."

Think of other ways to make your environment lead you toward, rather than away from, your goals. Eat your favorite snack while working on your most detested study material. Place a study review card on your car seat at the end of the day. In the morning, as you pick it up, keep it handy to look at during the red lights or while stuck in traffic. Be consistent and use whatever works for you.

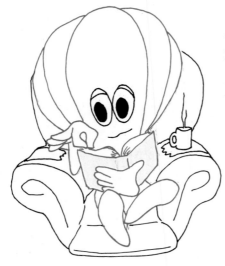

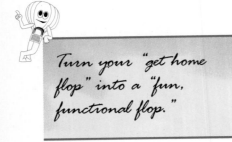

Turn your "get home flop" into a "fun, functional flop."

Note-Taking Strategies

Research demonstrates that the color yellow seems to enhance memory. Use yellow notepaper or yellow index cards for class notes, and yellow highlighters for marking important passages in textbooks or as you review your class notes. If you need a second color, either for variety or for contrasting concepts, consider using lime-green. This color, too, has been found to enhance memory.

As mentioned before, it is best to use yellow index cards (4 × 6 inches or 3 × 5 inches). Give each card a major heading (such as "left heart failure"). This makes it easier to flip back to the card to add information if the teacher wanders among topics. You might want to further divide one or more cards by subheadings of the nursing process (such as "left heart failure, interventions"). Carry a few cards with you at all times. In idle times, such as waiting in a drive-through or waiting to pick the children up after school, these cards will be a lifesaver in terms of making use of your time. And with more frequent exposure to content, the difficulty level of the material will seem to decrease.

How do you learn? Is there an easiest or best way? Is it by listening or by writing? Is it by looking at diagrams of the parts, then the whole? Is it by tasting? Which of your senses serve you the best as you strive for effective and efficient study techniques?

People usually have one sense or one style that serves them the best. You might determine what yours is by formal testing or just by listening to yourself and others in daily conversations:

Learning styles send you safe recall. Stimulate them.

- "You're not seeing what I'm saying." (Speaker uses a visual style.)
- "You're not hearing what I'm saying," (Speaker prefers a more verbal style.)
- "You're not feeling what I'm trying to say." (Speaker's style is more tactile.)
- Persons who feel most comfortable writing and taking notes are depending on more than hearing; they are also using the tactile and visual senses.
- Persons who draw pictures on their notes are using the visual style of learning or stimulation for recall.

One style is no better than another. The use of a combination of styles has been shown to enhance memory and recall of information. So be creative! Trash the traditional outline technique if you feel it's

Valuable memorization occurs as you make your audiotape. By the time your tape is made, you're already halfway there!

never worked for you. Try new note-taking techniques to see which one works best for you.

AUDIOTAPE CLASS LECTURES

Some schools have specific rules regarding the audiotaping of lectures. Be sure to get the permission of the instructor before taping. Plans are provided here for creating two types of audiotapes as study aids: the *structured* and *unstructured* self-audiotapes.

The Structured Self-Audiotape

Get some 90-minute audiotapes, which cost about the same as 60-minute audiotapes. The basic structure outline that follows will take up about 15 minutes of audiotape:

- Tape one minute of a piece of favorite music (choose something that makes you feel good or that puts you in a good mood). Dub in a 15-minute segment of study material. Then dub in more music for about 5 minutes after the segment. Make this music fit the mood or personality of the material you are reviewing.
- Continue filling the tape with 15-minute segments of material followed by 5-minute music segments.

Listening to this type of audiotape will easily fit into your schedule, like those 15-minute trips to the store. You can stop the tape and come back to it without the problem of starting in the middle of the material. If you do more 5- or 10-minute trips in the car, change the content time to reflect this.

The music interspersed throughout the tape will allow you time to relax and enhance your chances of remembering and associating the material, especially the more difficult content.

Be sure to keep each 15 minutes of material as a self-contained unit. One example of a congestive heart failure (CHF) outline for a self-audiotape is as follows:

- One minute of music
- Fifteen minutes for overview of the heart's circulation, reasons for failure, and medications given to treat and prevent failure
- Five minutes of music
- Fifteen minutes about left-sided heart failure (Do it first since the left heart function is the most important.) Here's the order I would suggest:
    1. Predisposing factors
    2. Comparison of acute and chronic findings, if pertinent
    3. Plans for home care (fluids, diet, exercise, and coping resources for stress, medications)
    4. Interventions for acute/home care follow-up
    5. Evaluation for effectiveness of specific medications given in the acute or chronic situation and therapies
    6. What changes need to be reported
- Five minutes of music
- Fifteen minutes right-sided heart failure (Use the same outline as with left heart failure.)
- Five minutes of music
- Fifteen minutes on other considerations (If you initially studied adult clients with heart failure, in this last segment you could add information about pediatrics and maternity considerations that are pertinent to heart failure.) Examples include the following:
    - Differences in findings (for example, for children versus adults, for pregnant women, high-risk pregnant women, or for patients with Type I or Type II diabetes)
    - Differences in interventions or therapies (for example, fluids, diet, exercise, coping resources, and medications)
    - Differences in teaching techniques based on

The structured outline for an audiotape

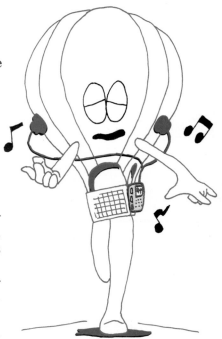

developmental or age considerations, physical attributes, financial concerns, and home environment
- Five minutes of music
- Three- to 5-minute summary
- End with music

Benefits In Using the Above Outline

In most cases, to follow this outline, you will have to repeat some material three to five times. This is the number of repetitions that the average person needs to remember information. You can select what to repeat according to the topic. Base this decision on what material you have trouble remembering.

Benefits In the Use of Music

Music interspersed with difficult material allows time to relax, and the musical association encourages recall. You can change the type of music from segment to segment if it will help you to remember. For example, I would use a fast-paced music for material on left heart failure and slower-paced music for right heart failure (which is more often insidious and slow).

Benefits of the Structured Self-Audiotape

These tapes can be used throughout school, added to, then used again for review and preparation for the licensing exam. The 15-minute segments can easily be taped over as you add to your knowledge base of specific pathologic conditions.

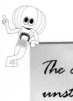

The content of an unstructured audiotape

The Unstructured Self-Audiotape

As you review your lecture notes, audiotape yourself as you read or make comments about the notes.

Limit this material to 15-minute segments. Tape music in between the segments, just as in the structured audiotape. Later, listen to this tape in the car or while you take a walk.

Audiotape a discussion of that "hard-to-remember material" with a friend. (Give the friend a copy of the tape.) Listen to it at your leisure.

Benefits of the Unstructured Self-Audiotape

These audiotapes can be re-recorded after each test or when you have a grasp of the material. These audiotapes are easy to make by recording as you think or read aloud. Your family's comments, taped between segments, can be a welcome assist when you get tired of studying. Ask friends or loved ones to say a few words of encouragement, or tell you why you are important. This may be just what you need to hear later when you're having a difficult day.

STORYTELLING, IMAGERY, AND ASSOCIATION

Stories are the retaining walls for remembering the most difficult content.

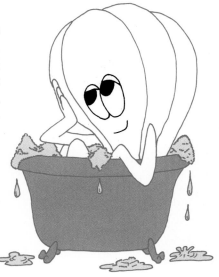

A creative, fun approach to memorization is to make up a story about the material that you want to recall. Associate the information with something you feel neutral or positive about, or something you might see or encounter every day. Make it simple, and make it fun! Coming up with crazy, unusual ideas will help you remember even better.

Have a friend make up a story about the same material; then share your stories, or maybe even combine them. Brainstorm about what kind of stories might fit different material during your down times (driving a car, sitting on the porch, taking a bubble bath, or whenever you are relaxed). The more you do it, the easier it will become. Ideas will pop into your mind! The following are just a few examples:

"Hyper" and "hypo" conditions: if you know one, then you know the other. Just think of the opposite.

Conditions That Are Opposites

For conditions and diseases that are "opposites," study one of them to know it thoroughly. Then tell yourself the other is the opposite.

For example, consistently study to know the "hyper" conditions, such as the effects of the sympathetic nervous system, or conditions like hyperthyroid, hyperglycemia, hyperparathyroid, hypertension, and Cushing's syndrome (hypersteroids). This gives your thinking process a pattern for learning new material that will enable you to retain and recall it more easily.

If a question asks about a "hypo" condition, list or recall what you know about the "hyper" condition. Then discern their opposites to reveal the "hypo" findings.

You may find it easier to consistently remember the "hypo" conditions. In that case, accept the "hyper" findings as opposite. The best method for you may depend on how you process information or what your life experiences are. For example, if you know someone who takes Synthroid, it may be easy for you to recall that it is critical to monitor for excess effects of the drug. This could be your springboard to remembering the "hyper" findings in various disease processes or drug effects.

The Sympathetic or Adrenergic System

I remember the sympathetic or adrenergic system by thinking of it as the brakes in a car: the use of it is limited. If a car's brakes are used excessively, they wear out. The same thing happens to a body with excessive sympathetic stimulation.

Read over the sympathetic stimulation findings listed in Table 7-1. Then fill in the *overstimulation* of

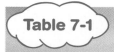 Table 7-1	**Sympathetic Stimulation and Parasympathetic Overstimulation**	
Body System	**Sympathetic Stimulation**	**Parasympathetic Overstimulation (Fill In by Thinking of Opposite)**
Pupils	Dilation	
Nose/mucous membranes	Dry from vasoconstriction	
Lungs	Bronchodilation	
Heart	Increased heart rate, increased contractility, dilation of the coronary arteries	
Pancreas	Increased insulin, increased glucagon	
Liver	Increased formation of glucose	
Gallbladder	Nothing; no bile release	
GI tract	Decreased peristalsis, constipation	
Bladder	Decreased peristalsis, urine retention	

the parasympathetic or cholinergic findings by thinking of the opposite. (Note that I have also incorporated the use of a head-to-toe approach to help recall.)

Think of the parasympathetic system as having the functions of a parent. Just as parents regulate their children—making sure that they are properly bathed, dressed, and fed, tucked into bed at night and sent off to school in the morning—the parasympathetic system keeps bodily functions in check to prevent over- or under-functioning. Therefore, the parasympathetic (or cholinergic) system maintains our day-to-day bodily functions. It maintains or modulates the following parameters:

• Heart rate between 60 and 100 beats per minute

- Bowels on schedule
- The ability to take a deep breath or to sneeze
- Release of bile according to the ingestion of fat
- Body alertness to bladder function needs
- Mouth moistness

The Low Calcium Train Travels the Tracks

An express train engine, labeled "Low Calcium," pulls a car labeled T, a double-stacked car labeled TC and TT, and ends with another T car (see Figure 7-1). The fact that this is a speeding train signals that low calcium results in faster, tenser muscle motion. The Ts on the cars represent the findings of low calcium.

The T nearest the engine is the more common indicator of low calcium. This T equals tingling of the fingertips, tongue, lips, or brain (dizziness). These are the most common findings when people hyperventilate; they occur *not* because the serum level of calcium has dropped, but because normal calcium mechanisms are *hindered* when the body is in an alkalotic state such as that caused by hyperventilation.

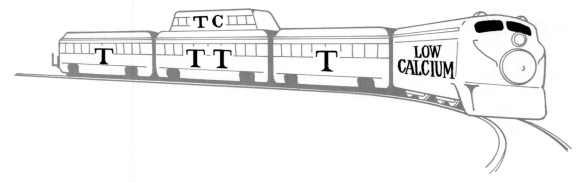

Figure 7-1   The Low Calcium Train travels the tracks.

What do TC and TT stand for? The first T in each set stands for twitching. The second letters, C and T, give clues about where to look or what to do. C stands for Chvostek's sign. Do this by tapping the cheekbone 1 to 2 inches in front of the ear. Look for twitching on the side of the mouth (if tapping on the right cheekbone, look for a twitch on the right side of the mouth; if tapping on the left cheekbone, look for a twitch on the left side of the mouth).

Next, T equals Trousseau's sign. To conduct this, place a tourniquet on either of the arms for about 1 minute, longer than you would if you were taking a blood pressure. Slowly release the pressure in the cuff, looking for a twitch or spasm in the fingers or wrist. A twitch in the fingers equals the extension of the fingers to where the tips come together. A twitch of the wrist equals flexion of the wrist.

The final T train car has a trail of darkness and gloom. This T equals tetany or tonic seizure activity, the most severe finding with low calcium.

Moral of the Low Calcium Train Story

In the story, the Low Calcium Train travels the two tracks with tonnage of the three Ts—Tingling; Twitching, both Chvostek's and Trousseau's signs; and Tetany. These muscle findings may result from one of two major reasons (like the two train tracks):

1. Low serum calcium levels
2. An interference with calcium metabolism, as in an alkalotic condition

The Low Calcium Train travels two tracks with the tonnage of three T cars.

If one of the three Ts is found to be present, and a serum calcium level is not available, check two items—the client's history and acid-base status—before an injection of calcium.

So, to recall the signs of low calcium, when you see a train or cross the train tracks, say:

- "T, TC and TT, T"; or else just stutter the Ts
- Or say, "Where's the calcium?"

Remember the opposite method discussed earlier? Use it here. A high calcium finding equals the opposite finding—degrees of muscle weakness to paralysis.

Minimal Magnetic Magnesium

Low magnesium has the same findings as found on the low calcium train. The most common clinical conditions with low serum magnesium levels are preeclampsia, eclampsia, acute myocardial infarction, and post open heart surgery. Magnesium can be given within a safer margin of error—normal levels are 1.5 to 2.5 mEq/L. Significant clinical findings are typically not evident until serum levels exceed 8 or 9 mEq/L.

OVERCOMING MENTAL BLOCKS DURING CLASS OR EXAMS

Mental blocks happen when you seek an immediate answer in a direct, linear way, yet your brain needs time to free-associate for the solution. With the left brain being more "fact friendly" and the right brain more "idea friendly," both sides interact in a complementary way to come up with creative solutions to problems.

So how can you use this hemispheric control to overcome mental blocks? Simply start scribbling or manipulating a small object with your other hand. This triggers the non-dominant side of your brain to do things it normally doesn't do. The unfamiliar muscular movements from the non-dominant side of your body will trigger new thoughts from the non-dominant side of your brain. This gives you some

If you're stuck, use your other hand.

fresh insights. Historically, Leonardo da Vinci and Benjamin Franklin both advocated the use of the non-dominant hand to find additional answers.

Determine Your Brain/Body Dominance

Take a trip from head to toe to determine the dominance or non-dominance of your body sites. Once you know the dominant way you move, break out of mental blocks by activating non-dominant body parts.

Eyes: We typically focus on an object with one eye, instead of both eyes. To determine which eye is dominant, simply hold your thumb out at arm's length in front of you, using it to block out a small object on the far wall (such as a light switch or the corner of a picture frame). Do this with both eyes open. Now close your right eye. If your thumb is still blocking out the object, then your left eye was dominant in focusing. If you can see the object beside your thumb, then you focused on it with your right eye.

Wink: Wink one eye, then the other. Does winking one eye feel more natural than the other? If so, that is your dominant eye for winking.

Smile: Smile into a mirror. Which side of your mouth goes higher? Which side of your face has more wrinkles? That side is your dominant one.

Arms: Cross your arms with one arm on top of the other. Whichever one is on top is the dominant one.

Thumbs: Bring your hands together, interlocking your fingers, making sure you have one thumb on top of the other. Whichever thumb is on top is your dominant thumb. Now, separate your hands and bring them back together with the other thumb on top. Feels awkward, doesn't it?

Hands: Are you right-handed or left-handed?

Wink when you are weary. It relaxes the mind's eye and the muscles of the eye, and it exercises the facial muscles.

Use a head-to-toe approach to determine your body and brain dominance.

Legs: Cross your legs at the knees. Which leg feels more comfortable on the top? That's your dominant leg.

Thinking gestures: This exercise requires the help of another person. Have a friend ask you a question, then observe whether your eyes move to the left or the right as you contemplate the answer. Do not stare at each other; your eyes need to be relaxed to move. If your eyes go up and down *before* they go to the side, that's natural. Your eyes normally go *up* when you are *visualizing* the answer to a question like "What was I wearing last Tuesday?" Your eyes normally go *down* when you are *feeling* the answer to a question like "Was the ocean cold that day?" If your eyes don't move to one side or the other, allow yourself to be observed later at a more spontaneous time. Note if your eyes move to the right or the left. This, too, is a sign of brain dominance.

Visualization: Close your eyes and visualize a circular clock on the wall in front of you. Imagine reaching out to take the clock off the wall and put it on the front of your face. Now put one finger of one hand at 12 o'clock and one finger of the other hand at 3 o'clock. Open your eyes and note if 3 o'clock is on the right or left side of your face. Mark down which side (Thompson, 1992).

Score Your Dominance

Count the number of right- and left-sided dominances you have (for example, seven for the right side and three for the left side). These body dominances show the *exact opposite* brain dominance since the left side of the body is controlled by the right side of the brain and vice versa.

What Does This Mean to You?

If you get stuck during study, review, or testing, simply do something to stimulate the non-dominant side

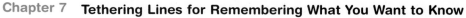

of your brain. Some techniques to do this include the following:

- Cross your legs the "wrong" way.
- Interlock your fingers the "wrong" way.
- Use your non-dominant eye to read the content or question.
- Write down thoughts with your non-dominant hand.
- Doodle or scribble with the "wrong" hand.
- Breathe through your left nostril for a right-brain jolt.
- Breathe through your right nostril for a left-brain jolt.

The unfamiliar stimulates new thoughts for problem solving.

Do you have a desire to achieve a better balance in your brain dominance? Here are some suggestions for things to do if you are *left* brain dominant:

- Fly a kite.
- Learn to dance.
- Take a course in storytelling.
- Find a way to be with and play with children.
- Draw.
- Paint.
- Use colored pencils and pens for note-taking.

Here are some suggestions to stimulate the left side of the brain if you are *right* brain dominant:

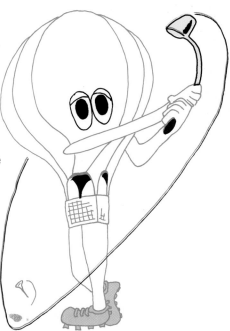

- Make miniature models.
- Start some type of collection (for example, baseball cards or stamps).
- Keep a daily checkbook balance to the penny.
- Keep dated records of your activities.
- Play golf, bridge, or chess.

- Read history or science books.
- Take up ballroom dancing (Thompson, 1992).

SUMMARY

The study strategies discussed in this chapter moved from general study tips to focus on the keys to effective note-taking and audiotaping. We looked at associations, imagery, and storytelling, and offered tips on overcoming mental blocks by harnessing brain dominance.

Research has shown that the colors yellow and, to a lesser extent, lime green can enhance memory skills. Note-taking with yellow index cards and highlighters can help in stimulating memory and recall.

The use of short segments of key material interspersed with personal music choices makes both structured and unstructured self-audiotapes effective lines of memory and recall. Both storytelling and mental imagery can help you associate symbols with key facts for ease in recall.

Finally, engaging in exercises to familiarize yourself with your own brain dominance can help you overcome mental blocks. Whenever you are stuck, simply use a movement that stimulates the nondominant side of your brain to get new insights for problem resolution.

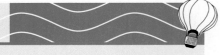

Air Currents

"Writing down your ideas is like money in the bank."

Charles "Chic" Thompson

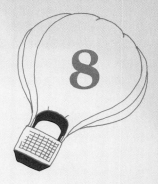

Maneuvering Metaphors to Recall Lab Values

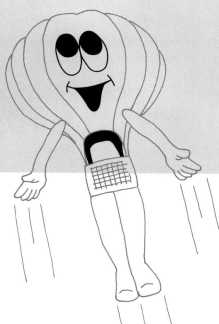

"Imagine your brain as a block of wax with thoughts imprinted into it."

Plato

Just as an aeronaut, or balloonist, must be aware of measures associated with ideal flight conditions (wind velocity, altitude, and calculating fuel needs), so the test-taker preparing for exams must be able to recall key lab values. It doesn't take very many of these before the most avid memorizer feels overwhelmed. Is there any way to increase your power to recall numbers?

Chapter 7 discusses the use of storytelling and imagery to create associations that aid memory. Similarly, an easy way to recall a lot of numbers is through the use of metaphors. A metaphor connects two different universes of meaning through some similarity they share. Metaphors help us understand one idea by means of another. The key to metaphor-

> ### Box 8-1
>
> ## *Two Kinds of Thinking*
>
> **HARD THINKING**
> - Logical, precise, exact, specific, consistent
> - Focusing on the differences among things
> - "Spotlight" thinking: bright, clear, intense with a narrow focus used when you want to "get something done"
> - Used most commonly during test situations to evaluate information, narrow the options, and make a decision
>
> **SOFT THINKING**
> - Metaphorical, approximate, humorous, playful
> - Focuses on the similarities and connections among things
> - "Floodlight" thinking: softer, diffuse, less intense and with a wider focus
> - Used when you want to be "thinking something different"
> - Used more commonly during study and review of content to search for new ideas for recall of difficult content, to think globally, and to manipulate problems
> - Might be used after you have narrowed the options to two for a decision of which option is the best

Adapted from Roger von Oech.

"The metaphor is probably the most fertile power possessed by man."

Jose Ortega Y Gasset

"There are two kinds of people in this world: those that divide everything into two groups, and those that don't."

Kenneth Boulding

ical thinking is similarity; this is often how our thinking ability can be expanded.

Metaphorical thinking is sometimes thought of as an example of "soft" thinking. "Soft" thinking has a broad focus and reveals the *similarities* among things. "Hard" thinking examines the *differences* among things and has a narrow focus. Both types of thinking are useful as you study, review, and take exams (see Box 8-1).

Metaphors are effective in making complex content easier to understand. The Bible is often metaphorical; refer to the Book of Proverbs for excellent examples of the use of metaphorical thinking.

Some great examples of everyday metaphorical thinking are all around us. For instance, we say that hammers have "heads," tables have "legs," roads have "shoulders," and beds have "feet." Can you think of more examples? Challenge yourself to identify when you or those around you are speaking or thinking in metaphors. Then apply them to make number values—particularly lab values—meaningful. The following examples of how to recall lab values more easily are based on metaphorical thinking. Use them as a springboard for launching others of your own.

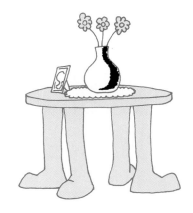

WHAT ARE THE BEST YEARS OF YOUR LIFE?

Many people say that the best years of your life are from **35** to **45** years of age. By this time, for most of us, our youthful struggles, and those of our children, are beginning to subside, yet we are young enough and healthy enough to take on new challenges. You don't buy that? Well, for the purposes of this memory exercise, just accept it: the most functional years of your life are from 35 to 45.

Now look at these serum lab values. Remember: the best years of your life are **35** to **45** years of age.

- Normal pH acid-base range = 7.**35** to 7.**45**
- Normal CO_2 (carbon dioxide) range = **35** to **45**
- Normal Na (sodium) range = **135** to **145**
- Normal K (potassium) range = **3.5** to **4.5** (Actually it is 5.0, but 4.5 is close enough to get you to the correct answer. *Don't forget the decimal*—otherwise, the client will be dead with potassium levels of 35 to 45. Remember that

Remember 35-45 and you will have memorized the values of four key lab tests.

when cells die or necrose, potassium is released, resulting in a higher potassium level for 48 to 72 hours.)

However—

- Normal HCO_3^- (bicarbonate) values can be thought of as symbolized by that period in which you *think* it is the best years of your life: 22 to 26!
- Exception to this thought: The normal CO_2 range = *50 to 60 for people with chronic lung disease.*

HOW OLD WILL YOU LIVE TO BE?

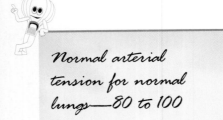

Normal arterial tension for normal lungs—80 to 100

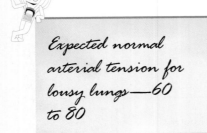

Expected normal arterial tension for lousy lungs—60 to 80

Normal PaO_2 = 80 to 100 (or, equal to the average number of years most people will live). Most of the people in this age group (80-100) will be **S**ingle without a **S**pouse on a **Sat**urday night. So 80 to 100 = normal arterial O_2 **Sat**uration.

However, some people have lousy lungs from chronic lung disease. The average years most of these lousy lung people will live equals 60 to 80 = the normal PaO_2 for them. If these clients have a PaO_2 >80, the respirations may be dramatically slowed or stopped.

Recall tip: These individuals usually have a higher respiratory rate to begin with. Their respiratory rate is usually in the mid to high 20s. Usually they use accessory muscles. Thus if their PaO_2 >80, their respiratory rate may drop to 16 from 28, which is a significant finding for these clients.

The average period in years for more complications of people with chronic lung disease equals the mid to high 50s and 60s = normal $PaCO_2$ range for people with chronic lung disease. Associate CO_2 levels (50s to 60s) with ages for **c**omplications for **c**hronic lung **c**onditions. *Their respiratory drive changes from responding to high levels of $PaCO_2$ to responding to lower levels of PaO_2 (<80) since the $PaCO_2$ is chronically elevated.*

Usually, no difference exists in arterial O_2 saturation for people with chronic lung disease: **Sat**uration = 80 to 100 = the same arterial O_2 saturation expected for all people.

GROWING UP

Siblings

Normal magnesium (Mg) = **1.5-2.5** mEq/L
Normal potassium (K) = **3.5-5** mEq/L

Consider K and Mg as siblings in the same family. When one sibling does an action, the other repeats it. So it is with K and Mg. When K is lost and low in the serum, usually so is Mg, and vice versa. Magnesium has an "n" in it; thus its value is "not" as much as that for K. More exactly, normal Mg is half as much as normal K. Similarly, a younger sibling (Mg, who comes later in the alphabet) might be only half as big as an older brother or sister.

Females and Males

Normal hematocrit (Hct) = **35-45%** (the best years of life)
Normal hemoglobin (Hgb) = **12-16** g/dl **for females**
Normal hemoglobin (Hgb) = **14-18** g/dl **for males**

Contrast the developmental processes of teenagers. Girls mature earlier than boys. Therefore, females have lower normal hemoglobin than males.

Fuel for the Fun

A third consideration in growing up is the need for glucose, which typically enters the bloodstream through the gastrointestinal (GI) tract. Glucose is the essential fuel for the brain, where fun activities are thought of. If glucose is unavailable via the GI tract, the body will produce it by one of two ways:

- The breakdown of glycogen stores in the liver
- The breakdown of the body's muscle mass

Glucose is checked and monitored by these tests:

Random glucose—varies with time of test/last meal

Fasting glucose—70 to 110 mg/dl typically taken in the morning with no ingestion of food or fluids except water after midnight

Glucose tolerance test—the definitive test for diabetes mellitus and gestational diabetes

One hour post–50 g oral glucose—initial screening test for gestational diabetes with pregnant women at 24 to 28 weeks

Hgb A_{1C}—screening test for the average glucose over a prior period of 2 to 3 months; requires no special preparation; can be obtained immediately after eating or insulin administration; at risk over 8.8%, which indicates recent hyperglycemia

COUNT ON YOUR FINGERS AND THUMBS FOR CLOTTING

The two drugs for anticoagulation (that is, for *prevention,* not dissolution, of clots) are the following:

- Heparin, which is given SQ or IV
- Coumadin, which is given PO only

If a clot is to be dissolved, the term is *lysis*. Medications for lysis (for example, Activase) are more commonly tested on advanced content exams.

Now get your fingers and thumbs ready! Hold all of them up and out, and follow these directions:

Heparin

- Spell out the word h-e-p-a-r-i-n on your digits. Note that you have three digits left.
- Heparin counted on the fingers and thumb leaves three digits left over = PTT (partial thromboplastin time). This is the lab value to monitor heparin therapy.
- Also, associate the three fingers left over with the first number for a normal PTT (around 30 seconds). PTT is also written as aPTT or as activated partial thromboplastin time. *Therapeutic* lab levels are 1½ to 2 times normal (or a maximum of around 60 seconds).
- Also associate the three fingers left up with the initial time it takes heparin to be effective— usually within **30** minutes—and the fact that one dose lasts for around **3** hours).

Heparin—three fingers left = PTT = normal value around 30 seconds

Recall tip: Remember that the normal lab value is around 30 seconds. Use it as a basis to calculate the maximum therapeutic levels (1½ to 2 times normal). Read the question precisely! Is the question asking for a *therapeutic* or a *normal* value for the PTT?

Warning! Therapeutic levels are different from normal levels.

Coumadin

- Spell out the word C-o-u-m-a-d-i-n on your digits. Note that you have two digits left.
- Associate these two digits left over with PT (prothrombin time). This is the lab test to monitor Coumadin therapy.
- Also associate the two fingers left over with the

Coumadin—two fingers left = PT = normal value is up to 20 seconds

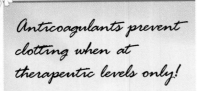

Anticoagulants prevent clotting when at therapeutic levels only!

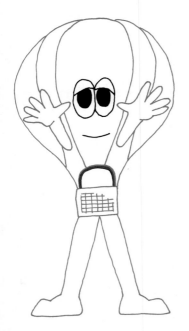

first number for a *normal* PT, which equals around 20 seconds (in some labs 15 to 20 seconds). *Therapeutic* lab levels equal 1½ to 2 times normal (or a maximum of around 40 seconds).

- Also associate the two fingers left over with the time it takes Coumadin, only given PO, to be effective or therapeutic (usually within 2 days [48 to 72 hours]). And recall the fact that once stopped, Coumadin has effects for 7 to 10 days or 2 weeks over which time bleeding precautions are taken.

Recall tip: Remember the normal lab value of 15 to 20 seconds. Use it as a basis to calculate the maximum therapeutic levels (1½ to 2 times normal). Again, read the question precisely! Is the question asking for a *therapeutic* or a *normal* value?

ON THE COUNT OF 10

Associate your 10 digits with the following crucial normal values:

- BUN (blood urea nitrogen) = 10 to 20
- Calcium = 10
- Central venous or right atrial pressure = 10 (cm H_2O, as measured by a water manometer)
- Creatinine = 1.0 (think of it as a 10 with a decimal point after the 1)
- Hemoglobin A_{1C} = no greater than 10%
- Intracranial pressure = 10 (as measured by mm Hg)
- Urine specific gravity = 1.020 (think of it as 10-20 with a decimal point after the one)
- WBC (white blood cell) = 10,000 maximum and 5,000 minimum
  Leukocytosis = WBC >10,000
  Leukopenia = WBC <5,000

On the count of 10 think of these normal values.

LIFE IN LIVER CITY

In Chapter 7, storytelling metaphors were discussed. Figure 8-1 is a drawing of the liver. Now it's your turn to make up a story about life in "Liver City." The story should illustrate the functions of the liver and the lab tests that are used to evaluate them. This imaginative exercise might help you remember how the liver works. When you've finished, compare my Liver City (Figure 8-2) with yours!

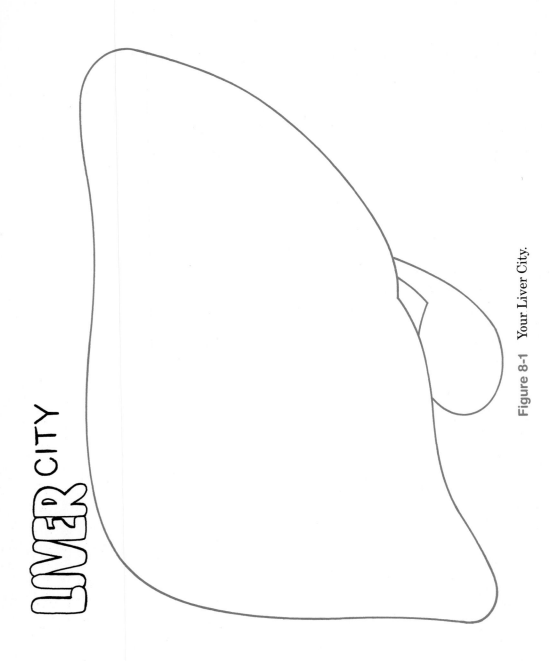

Figure 8-1 Your Liver City.

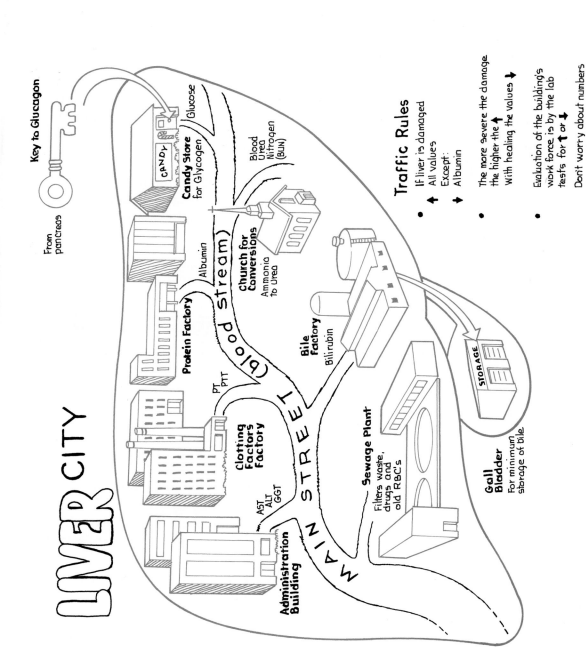

Figure 8-2   My Liver City.

> *"Without this playing with fantasy no creative work has ever yet come to birth. The debt we owe to the play of imagination is incalculable."*
>
> Carl Gustav Jung

SUMMARY

The calculation and recall of laboratory values is essential to basic nursing, just as values relating to velocity, altitude, and fuel needs are essential to ballooning. Typically, increases in laboratory values reflect an over-functioning or damaged organ. Decreases in values usually suggest a hypofunction of the related system. (Some exceptions to these generalizations exist. For example, an increase in the PTT indicates a lesser functioning of the liver.)

Relating an organ function to some aspect of life familiar to you can be one key to retaining lab values in your memory. The goal of any practitioner is to associate clinical findings to abnormal lab values with appropriate follow-up actions and the evaluation of therapy.

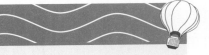

Air Currents

> *"Make friends with your shower. If inspired to sing, maybe the song has an idea in it for you."*
>
> Albert Einstein

> *"If at first you don't succeed, take a break."*
>
> Charles "Chic" Thompson

Lift-Off: It's Time for Critical Thinking

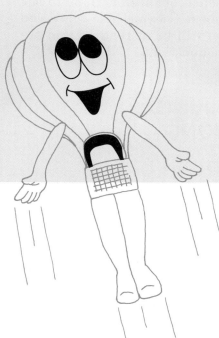

"Every child is an artist. The problem is how to remain an artist after growing up."

Pablo Picasso

For every aeronaut, the day comes when practice and checking equipment and flight calculations must end and the time for the first solo flight arrives. The pilot will now encounter a number of surprises that, it is hoped, will enable him or her to make creative decisions.

This is critical thinking time.

Chapters 7 and 8 featured a number of study strategies for memorization. But eventually, the time comes to sit down in the actual exam room, and the time for memorization will be over. What strategies are available to help you then? Inevitably, many questions will require more of you than simple recall of facts or lab values. These questions will require *critical thinking*. Although this makes them *sound* like harder questions, the *implementation* of critical thinking actually makes test-taking *easier*. This chapter shows you how, and it just may be the most important chapter in this book.

How do we implement critical thinking to aid in decision-making? First of all, a frequent error of test-takers with multiple-choice questions is reading the question incorrectly. The first and best piece of advice to take into a multiple-choice exam is to simply *read the question critically*! Learn to slow down and analyze the question by trying one or more of the following strategies. Do each of these actions to see which of them works best for you. The more you practice, the better you will be at reading and answering multiple-choice questions.

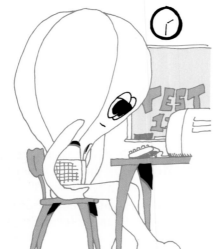

Read the question critically!

CRITICAL THINKING/ READING ACTIONS

Action 1: Slow Down Your Coordination

Slow your hands down to match the speed of your mind by sitting on both hands. After you have read all of the words in the stem and options, allow only one hand up to answer the question. Push the key on the computer keyboard with your *non-dominant* hand. Both of these actions will slow you down so you can make a conscious effort to read methodically. Using your non-dominant side also stimulates the opposite side of your brain for critical thinking and problem solving.

Action 2: Look Away and Breathe

Once you have made a decision, look away from the question. Take a slow, deep breath as you concen-

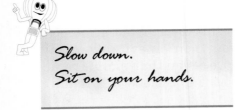

Slow down. Sit on your hands.

trate on your breath. Return to the test. Read the question with the intention of picking up new clues. Next, read your selected answer with this same intention. Go with your initial choice if new information isn't found.

Action 3: Draw a Picture of the Situation

You can do this in your mind by closing your eyes for a few seconds to picture the scene.

You can also do it on paper (*print* key words, do not write in cursive). Connect associated items with lines or directional arrows.

Draw a picture, either in your mind or on paper.

Action 4: Reword the Question

Reword the question in the format of subject, verb, object. Leave out any extraneous words.

State the question in your own words.

Action 5: Use the Eight Keys to Unfreeze Your Thinking

Key 1. With every reading of the question, be alert to key words such as the following:

- Most, least
- First, initially, immediately
- Best, main
- Short, long
- Toxic versus therapeutic levels
- Side effect versus expected effects versus toxic effects
- Complications of therapy versus complications of disease
- Usual problem versus unexpected problem

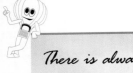

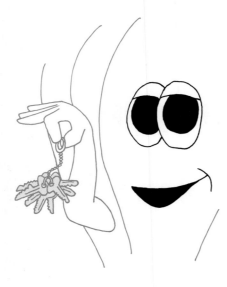

There is always a key to unlock your thinking.

- Most likely, commonly, frequently
- Be avoided
- In addition to

Key 2. Identify what nursing process step is being tested (assessment, analysis, planning, intervention, or evaluation).

Key 3. Make a note of time parameters. Examples include the following:

- Day one versus day three
- Preoperative
- Postoperative
- During
- After
- Before, prior to
- First, second, or third trimester; or first, second, or third stage of labor
- Time parameter versus a drug's initial onset of action versus peak action
- Early, late, terminal, frequency
- Predisposing condition versus complication

Key 4. Note unfamiliar words. Then reword the question without these words.

Key 5. Note the age of clients. Age groups are usually focused by decades (for example, 20s, 30s, 40s) for the developmental needs or the normal physiological aging, except for the first year of life. Each age group has different teaching needs as influenced by mental capabilities and physiologic functions, whether normal or abnormal (such as poor eyesight or the presence of illness). What is the client's functional mobility? Is there any history of strokes, weakening, or musculoskeletal injury? What is the degree of interest in information or in the presence of support systems?

Key 6. Identify words of essence such as "acute" versus "chronic" versus "terminal" or "partial" versus "total removal." Associate diseases that indicate an acute or chronic condition.

Key 7. Pinpoint locations such as the following:

- Hospital
- Outpatient center
- Home
- Extended care facility
- Postanesthesia unit
- Intermediate care facility

Key 8. Look for distractors. Popular examples of distractors are mystery diseases (strange illnesses that you have never heard of) or absurd conditions (such as "client walked in the hall naked"). Another type of distractor is any content that clashes with your personal beliefs or experience. You will know this occurs when you have an emotional reaction or response and your thinking becomes clouded and muddled.

Turn in your hunting license if you are quick on the trigger to react to distractors. Such actions can be fatal.

Finally, distractors can include emergency words that don't count when connected to more important words. Some emergency words are the following: *bright red, sanguinous,* and *bloody.* Consider this phrase: "Small amount of bright red blood." The amount is more important than the color, which serves mainly to distract you from what the question is really about. Other distracting emergency words include *edema* and *swelling.* Swelling in the neck is a greater threat because of the airway than swelling in the forearm. The site of swelling and the time involved are more critical than the fact that there is swelling.

PRACTICE QUESTIONS TO CLARIFY THE QUESTION

It's now time to practice the critical thinking/reading skills outlined above. The following are typical multiple-choice test questions you will have to answer on many of your tests:

1. During the assessment of a client with early left ventricular heart failure, the nurse might expect the client to report which of these findings?

2. In clients with sickle cell anemia, what terminal complication does the nurse anticipate if the sickling process occurs?

3. For the client with which diagnosis is the nurse most likely not to avoid instruction that includes the use of aspirin?

4. Which body system is unaffected by the enzymes given to children with cystic fibrosis?

5. In performing the assessment of this client, what should the nurse include to omit?

Now, reword each question in the space provided:

1. _____
_____
2. _____
_____
3. _____
_____
4. _____
_____
5. _____
_____

Finally, write down the actions or keys that you used to clarify the question:

1. _____
_____
2. _____
_____
3. _____
_____
4. _____
_____
5. _____
_____

DISCUSSION OF THE ACTIONS THAT COULD BE USED

Question 1: During the assessment of a client with early left ventricular heart failure, the nurse might expect the client to report which of these findings?
Key words include the following:

- "Early"—Look for findings such as shortness of breath (SOB) increased with exercise or at rest; and a dry, frequent cough. Don't be tricked into suggesting a congested chest or productive sputum, which are later findings of heart failure.
- "**L**eft"—Think **l**ung findings.
- "Client to report"—Match the education level, if given, with the level of words used.

Draw a picture:

- Make a drawing of the heart's chambers. Remember to contrast the right and left sides of the heart's physiology. The left heart chambers should be larger than the right heart chambers.

Nursing process step:

- Assessment.

Question 2: In clients with sickle cell anemia, what terminal complication does the nurse anticipate if the sickling process occurs?
Key words include the following:

- "Terminal"—At the end phase of a process.
- "Complications"—Undesired effects, not the predisposing factors of sickle cell anemia or the sickling process.

Time:

- "Sickling process occurs"—Recall that sickling results in clumping of red blood cells.

Reworded question:

- When sickling occurs, what is the complication that occurs at the end?

Question 3: For the client with which diagnosis is the nurse most likely not to avoid instruction that includes the use of aspirin?
Key words include the following:

- "Most likely"—These words have the highest priority.
- "Not to avoid"—Means you *would include* in the instruction.

Reworded question:

- For the client with which diagnosis is the nurse most likely to instruct about aspirin?

Question 4: Which body system is unaffected by the enzymes given to children with cystic fibrosis?
Key words include the following:

- "Unaffected"—Caution: read too quickly, this can be misread as "affected."

Reworded question:

- Which body system is not affected by the enzymes given to children with cystic fibrosis?

Question 5: In performing the assessment of this client, what should the nurse include to omit?

Reworded question:

- In performing the assessment of this client, what should the nurse omit?

SUMMARY

You may have to fly solo in an exam, but you needn't feel you have to navigate without tools. The first of these tools is to make yourself simply *slow down* as you *read the question*. After you have made your choice, look away and take a breather before reviewing the question one more time.

Other actions include drawing pictures, rewording the question, and using the eight keys discussed in this chapter. These keys or clues include keeping an eye out for any of the following: key words, nursing process steps, time parameters, unfamiliar words, ages, words of essence, locations of care, and simple distractions.

The good news is that not all multiple-choice test questions will be difficult to comprehend. However, preparation to decipher those questions that are difficult will result in a higher test score and minimize your tension or fatigue during the test. Apply the critical thinking actions and keys discussed in this chapter to multiple-choice questions. First and foremost, remember: read the question.

> *"Imagination was given to man to compensate for what he is not. A sense of humor was provided to console him for what he is."*
>
> *Horace Walpole*

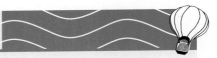

Air Currents

"Cultivate your imagination. Set aside time every day to ask yourself 'What if?' questions."

Charles "Chic" Thompson

"The thing always happens that you really believe in. And the belief in a thing makes it happen. And I think nothing will happen until you thoroughly and deeply believe in it."

Frank Lloyd Wright

"If you think you are beaten, you are; if you think you dare not, you don't; if you want to win, but think you can't, it's almost a cinch you won't. But, sooner or later, the man who wins is the man who thinks he can."

Author unknown

Handling the Ground Line for a Decision Between Two Options

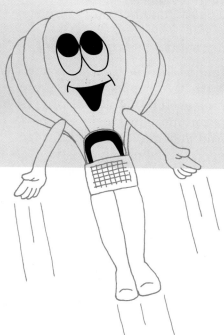

"The answers you get depend on the questions you ask."

Roger von Oech

Naturally, the last important step in flying well is *landing*! In fact, the pilot who can do everything else perfectly, but can't land, should not fly at all! The same is true of landing your final answer choice. No matter how strong your study, recall, reading, and analysis skills are, if you can't choose a final answer, you just might crash.

Does this scare you? Well, relax! If you can at least narrow the options from four to two, you've increased your odds of getting the correct answer from a 25% to a 50% chance! Once you reach this point, any of the six simple tips that follow can help you make the correct choice between two options.

TIP 1: CHANGE YOUR PROCESS OF READING

Most people repeatedly read the question, then the two options they think are the best choices. Do it differently.

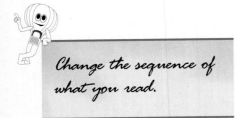
Change the sequence of what you read.

1. Read the question and note key words or clues.
2. Read one option and note key words or clues.
3. If you have made notes on scrap paper from other information in the stem, now is the time to review them.
4. Then read the question again.
5. Read the second option and note key words or clues.
6. Again refer to any notes on scrap paper.

The repeated reading of the question with each option provides you with two separate, complete thoughts. As you examine each thought, the mind is able to process information more precisely. You pick up on findings or words you may have otherwise missed. Try out this tip on the following question:

Sample Question

A young, pregnant client has a history of heroin addiction. For which of these problems should this client also be screened for a potential diagnosis at this time?

    a. Anemia
    b. Syphilis
    c. Tuberculosis
    d. Symptomatic bacteremia

Discussion

How do you narrow the options? Using the techniques covered in Chapter 9, most students should narrow the options to *b* and *c*. Options a and d are eliminated by the words "history of," information that indicates no present use of heroin.

Bacteremia is the presence of bacteria in the bloodstream. Anemia is the condition of having a lower than normal hemoglobin and hematocrit. Infection, such as bacteremia, would most likely come from dirty needles, and anemia could be caused by poor eating habits while using this drug.

Why are options b *and* c *better?* Options *b* and *c* may be findings of people with a history of heroin use. Sexually transmitted diseases, such as syphilis, may have occurred because the heroin user may perform sexual acts for money or in exchange for the drug. Tuberculosis (TB) occurs in drug users for numerous reasons, including the following:

- Poor living conditions
- Anorexia with improper food intake
- Exposure of the lung to the toxins of smoking

Finally, both conditions are more likely to linger after the addiction is broken, as opposed to anemia and bacteremia. Thus they are more consistent with a "history of" heroin addiction.

Now implement your new reading process: read the question and the first viable option, *b*; then the question and the second viable option, *c*.

> *b.* For which of these problems should this client also be screened for a potential diagnosis at this time? Syphilis
> *c.* For which of these problems should this client also be screened for a potential diagnosis at this time? Tuberculosis

You may have made either mental or written notes, such as the following:

- A pregnant client
- A "history of" heroin addiction

In reading the question the third time, most people would identify one or both of these clues:

- The time element: "at this time"
- The "potential diagnosis"

This guides you to think one step further. To definitively diagnose TB requires a sputum specimen to test for the acid-fast bacillus. No information is given that the client has a productive cough.

Do not get confused. The purified protein derivative test (PPD) is for screening (for a determination if someone has ingested the bacillus from *recent exposure to someone with active TB*). If the PPD is positive, then a chest x-ray is performed. On the other hand, to screen and diagnose syphilis in any stage requires a simple blood test, the rapid plasma reagin (RPR) test. Therefore the correct answer is option *b*.

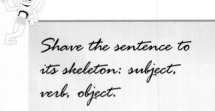

Shave the sentence to its skeleton: subject, verb, object.

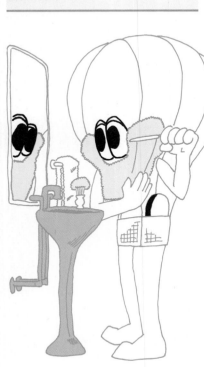

TIP 2: SHAVE OR SHORTEN THE SENTENCES

If the question or the options are lengthy, shave or shorten them to just *subject, verb, object*. Do this mentally or physically by writing the words down on a piece of scrap paper.

TIP 3: MAKE A REPORT

Make a written report from the given information. Make a note of these parameters on scrap paper just as you would if you were getting a verbal report at the change of shifts. These parameters might include such elements as:

- Time elements
- Degree of severity
- Internal or external elements
- Acute or chronic or terminal situation
- Specific or general tones to the situation
- Developmental status or age of client
- "History of" diseases or findings versus "acute" manifestations
- Findings associated with one another; groupings or patterns

Here's an example of how to look for groupings. Suppose the following information is given in the stem: ↑T (temperature), ↑HR (heart rate), and ↑R (respiration). Remember that an ↑T, especially >100, will ↑HR and ↑R. Avoid focusing on just the ↑R from the narrow application of the ABCS (airway, breathing, circulation, and safety)—with the airway and breathing being a priority. This will result in the narrow interpretation that respiration and airway are most important in this group of findings. Instead, reread the information, question, and options for clues to sort out what is the priority in the given situation.

Your notes should include information from the stem, the question, or the options as needed. Use abbreviations or symbols that you have used when you cared for clients. "An increased temperature of 102" looks different than "↑T 102." This helps your critical thinking abilities to implement a variety of skills such as the following:

- Quicker processing of material
- Quicker linking of related data
- Identifying of a pattern or grouping of data
- Seeing the whole picture
- Seeing the parts that make up the whole picture
- Seeing the relationship between various parts and between the parts and the whole picture

Make a report. If you have a mental block, write it out with your non-dominant hand. This stimulates the brain to see the information differently.

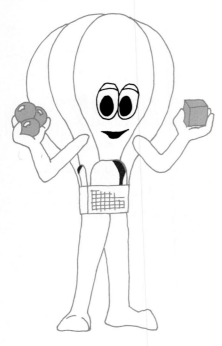

TIP 4: USE THE CLUSTER APPROACH ON THE OPTIONS

Use this approach if you have no idea of the correct answer:

1. Read all four options.
2. Reread the question.
3. Reread the options as you think of a theme to cluster or group three of the options under. For example:
   * Internal or external
   * Active or passive
   * Acute or chronic
   * Three options with any given organ or system, such as three options associated with the renal system and one with the cardiac system

The option that falls outside of the cluster—the odd one out—is more often than not the correct answer.

Try these tips on the question below.

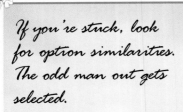

If you're stuck, look for option similarities. The odd man out gets selected.

Sample Question

An hour after receiving pain medication, a new post-operative client was still complaining of severe leg pain. The pain medication cannot be given again for another 2½ hours. How can the nurse best assist the client in dealing with the pain now?

a. Offer the client a magazine to read.
b. Guide the client in slow, rhythmic breathing techniques.
c. Turn the lights down low, give a PRN calming agent, and close the door.
d. Call the physician to ask for an increase in the dosage of the PRN pain medication.

Discussion

Did you use the approach of shaving the sentences down to subject, verb, and object? Do this either mentally or physically on paper for the stem:

"Client severe pain 1 hr after pain med. Nurse assists client now by?"

Now shave each option down to the following:

a. Offer magazine
b. Client breathes differently
c. ↓lights, give calming agent, close door
d. Call MD to ↑pain med

In the initial analysis of the four options, all of them look like good choices. You may have difficulty narrowing them down to two options.

Did you make notes as if getting a report with the application of your own knowledge? If you make a nursing report, one key word should have been identified: Severe!

Did you use the approach of clustering three options? Options *a, b,* and *c* can be clustered under the umbrella of "diversional approaches" to pain control. However, clients with severe pain after an operative procedure have a *physiological* need for pain control. Thus diversional therapy is not an effective choice to relieve such severe pain. Diversional therapies may be helpful for mild to moderate discomforts associated with some degree of emotional component. Pain medication is usually required for postoperative clients for 24 to 48 hours. This routine pain medication administration allows for easier movement and the promotion of deep breathing with the prevention of hypostatic pneumonia.

Clients with *severe* pain need to have it reported to the physician. Calming agents such as antianxiety or anxiolytics do nothing for severe physiologic pain. They may be helpful to minimize mild to moderate discomforts associated with emotional upset.

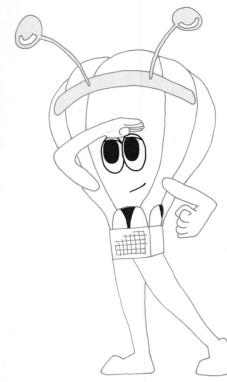

The correct answer is *d,* the only option not in the cluster related to diversional approaches to pain control.

TIP 5: BE ALERT WITH ANTENNAS UP IN YOUR COMFORT ZONES!

A graduate that I tutored stated at the beginning of a tutoring session: "I failed boards! I just missed it! In the report I can't believe that I did so poorly in the assessment area of the nursing process. I've been an LPN for 10 years, and I know my findings of the diseases."

This graduate had good reason to be astounded— what a puzzle! As the graduate worked on practice questions in my presence, I too observed that the graduate continually missed the assessment questions. I then had the graduate read the question and options out loud as we worked together on more questions.

Bingo! The graduate, on assessment questions, was reading some words incorrectly and accidentally changing the meanings of the stem or options— putting in *what was in the mind* instead of *what was on the paper.* For instance, the graduate might read "hypotension" as "hypertension," or "increase" as "decrease." Sometimes the graduate just added words that were not there.

Have you ever done this? Is it the result of nervousness? Not necessarily, although it can, of course, happen because of nervousness, tension, or fatigue. In this instance, it happened simply because the graduate had a comfort zone with certain material.

Is it good to have a comfort zone of knowledge? Yes, it is, just as it is good to feel comfortable driving down a familiar road. However, if you should drive in an unfamiliar place, you know you must pay more attention to the same old familiar task of driving. In the same

Comfort zones demand more energy and attention to ensure that what is on your mind is also what is on the paper or computer screen.

manner, use those same antennas or alerts with comfortable material in new or unfamiliar test situations.

How? First, identify the content in which you have a comfort zone. Then recognize those types of test questions during a test or during practice tests. Make sure that when you recognize comfort zone material, you *slow down* and read what is *on the page* and not *what is in your head*.

Make your initial choice of the best option. Then close your eyes and take a cleansing breath while you think of nothing. When you open your eyes, read just the question followed by the option you selected.

If you have misread as a result of familiarity, the rereading of the question and the selected option will usually help you to recognize any error. If you have made an error, start the rereading process of selection over with the remaining three options.

TIP 6: READ BACKWARDS, READ VERTICALLY

Once you have narrowed your answer to two options, as you read the question and option one then the question and option two (as in Tip 1), use a new sequence. Read the viable options from bottom to top (for example, *d* and *a,* or *c* and *b,* or *b* and *a*). This process clears your mind for better comprehension. Here's how this works:

> *Start with the bottom option and read up to the top option. Do this if you are nervous or stuck on two options.*

Sample Question

What observations are anticipated in a client who is hemorrhaging?

   a. Rising temperature, headache, weak pulse
   b. Shortness of breath, generalized discomfort, thready pulse

c. Hypertension, mottled skin, irregular pulse
    d. Sighing respirations, decreased urine output, a faster pulse

Discussion

First be alert to the fact that "hemorrhage" and "shock" questions are common comfort zone questions! How did you read the options? In a sequence of *a, b, c,* and then *d*? In other words, did you read all three items in each series for each option as you went from option *a* to option *d*?

Instead, read the first item only in each series from option *a* to option *d:* rising temperature, shortness of breath, hypertension, sighing respiration. Next, read the second item in each series from option *a* to option *d*. Then read the last item in each series from option *a* to option *d*.

If you read in the sequence of content presented in the options, you have an increased risk of misreading or glossing over key words. By altering the sequence as I've just described, you tend to experience better comprehension of the words and less misreading.

You may have narrowed the options to two at this point. Now read backwards within each option, reading the last item in the series, then the middle one, then the first item as indicated below:

- Option *d,* a faster pulse
- Option *c,* irregular pulse
- Option *b,* thready pulse
- Option *a,* weak pulse

Then read the middle item in each sequence:

- Option *d,* decreased urine output
- Option *c,* mottled skin
- Option *b,* generalized discomfort
- Option *a,* headache

Finally, read the first item in each sequence:

- Option *d,* sighing respirations
- Option *c,* hypertension
- Option *b,* shortness of breath
- Option *a,* rising temperature

Four common errors for these types of options with a series of items are:

1. To read "hypertension" as "hypotension" because that is what you are thinking of as you keep in mind that the client is hemorrhaging.
2. To gloss over "decreased urine output" since it is the *second item* in the series.
3. To *change the rules* for a correct option with a series—that two correct items out of three items in a series indicates a correct answer. The test-taker may select *b* because of "shortness of breath" and "thready pulse." Remember—all the items in a series must be correct. In this case, a client with hemorrhage may have generalized discomfort. However, that is too general of a finding and not the best choice.
4. To get stuck on the word "sighing" with an inability to associate it with a sigh or deep breath.

> *Common errors require full attention to convert them to uncommon errors.*

The correct answer to this question is option *d.* Now try these strategies on the question below:

Sample Question

The staff evaluates a neonate's function by Apgar parameters. All but which of these criteria should a staff member include?

a. Heart rate
b. Respiratory rate
c. Muscle tone
d. Reflex irritability

Discussion

Did you identify a comfort zone? Maybe you were tempted to make a knee-jerk choice or to apply the ABCS. Put your antennas up!

The most common errors with this type of question arise from the tendency to:

- Misread the question.
- Apply the wrong principle (the ABCS).
- Miss a key word by glossing over it. The key word in this question is a small one.
- Get stuck on the thought that *all* options are correct by reading the options in this manner: the heart, the lungs, the muscles, and the reflexes.

Do your "close eyes, deep breathing" exercise. Now reread the question and your selected option. Try rewording the question to: "Which of these criteria is not used with Apgar?" If you misread the question initially, you might have caught it by this point.

> *"The important thing, however, is to look for a second right answer, because unless you do, you won't find it."*
> Roger von Oech

What if you are stuck or still uncertain? To get unstuck, read the options backwards (from option *d* to option *a*) and put the last word in each before the first words:

d. Irritability of reflexes
c. Tone of the muscle
b. Rate of the respirations
a. Rate of the heart

If you're still not sure of the answer, think of the following:

- The reflexes are either "hypo" or "hyper"
- The tone is either flaccid or spastic
- The rate of the respirations—antennas up!

This is a newborn! What do you think? What else do you observe in newborns? Do grunting, sternal retractions, and nasal flaring mean anything to you? The rate of the heart should be 120 to 160. Notice that you could quickly come up with a parameter for all choices except the respirations of a neonate.

Yes! The correct answer is option *b.* Respiratory rate is not included in Apgar parameters.

What then is the respiration component of the Apgar parameters? It's respiratory *effort,* not *respiratory rate*! Also recall that a C-section neonate has a higher risk of respiratory difficulties because it doesn't travel through the birth canal, a process that squeezes fluid from the lungs. Therefore these neonates usually have initial findings of increased respiratory effort. However, do remember that abdominal breathing is expected in all neonates and is not a sign of respiratory distress.

SUMMARY

Relax! Work with these six tips as you do your practice exams. Make them as familiar to you as a good friend. They make a good ground line for "landing" a correct answer.

Tip 1: Change your process of reading.

Tip 2: Shave or shorten the sentences.

Tip 3: Make a written report.

Tip 4: Use the cluster approach on the options.

Tip 5: Be alert with antennas up in your comfort zones!

Tip 6: Read backwards, read vertically for options with a series of items.

"The only person who likes change is a wet baby."

Roy Blitzer

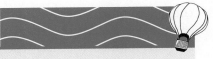

Air Currents

"Ideas are like rabbits. You get a couple, and learn how to handle them, and pretty soon you have a dozen."

John Steinbeck

"Genius is one percent inspiration and ninety-nine percent perspiration."

Thomas Alva Edison

"A professional is someone who can do his best work when he doesn't feel like it."

Alistair Cooke

11

Driving Style and Test-Taking Style: Prescriptive Actions

"The basic secret of overcoming worry is the substitution of faith for fear as your dominant mental attitude. Two great forces in this world are more powerful than others. One is fear and the other is faith. Faith is stronger than fear."

Norman Vincent Peale

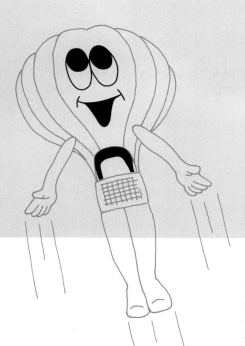

During every balloon trip a ground crew chases the balloon with two or more vehicles. The number of vehicles used depends on the number of persons in the balloon. A truck or van is typically necessary to take the repacked basket and balloon home with its owner.

Think of yourself as a balloon chaser and the driver of one vehicle. What is your style of driving? What is your style of planning and carrying out a trip? What if the trip is unexpected? What if unex-

What kind of driver are you?

What kind of test-taker are you?

Do you see any similar characteristics?

pected events occur? What if you get lost? What if you get anxious? Do your actions change? Your driving characteristics may be similar to your test-taking characteristics. By now you probably have identified some lapses in your test-taking or study skills. Let's look at some actions that you might take before or during a test. Then we will establish your style and give you some prescriptive actions for improving your test-taking skills. The prescriptive actions are all based on principles covered in this book.

THE SPEEDSTER

Directions: Check all that apply to you. During a test do you:

☐ Hurry through the entire test process in a desperate rush to finish before the facts are forgotten?

☐ Feel a racing pulse? Have rapid respirations?

☐ Feel neuromuscular excitement? Tremors? Twitching? Flushing?

☐ Misread, misinterpret, or mistake options because of your determination to get through the test?

☐ Have a tendency, when reading, to skip some of the words in the stem or options?

☐ Feel that you have to get done soon after the first few people complete the exam?

☐ Repeatedly read into the questions, options, or situations?

☐ Pore over "selected questions" with great intensity or concentration?

☐ Tend to overanalyze and lose sight of the actual intent of the given information, question, or options?

☐ Tend to have a knee-jerk reaction in deciding the correct answer?

☐ Select the "correct" option quickly by focusing on one word or part of the situation you perceive as critical without giving other words/events equal attention?

☐ When studying with others, think of what you are going to say next, instead of putting your mind into idle and listening to what others are saying or asking about the topic?

If you checked two or more of the above questions you are a *speedster*. You have a heavy foot on the gas pedal most of the time, and you need to:

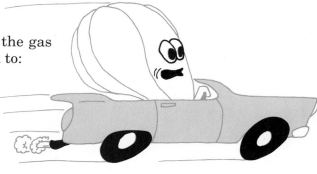

1. Develop a plan of test review.
2. Start reviewing for your tests at least 1 week before the test.
3. Schedule 15 minutes every day to read over your notes from your classes of that day.
4. Start a day early to "cram" for the exam rather than "cram" the night before.
5. Do at least five questions with the timer set for 5 minutes two to three times a week.
   a. Your goal is to have <2 minutes left on the timer.
   b. If you have >2 minutes left on the timer, you are going too fast. Slow down.
   c. Reset the timer for 5 minutes. Do five more questions as you attempt to slow down.
   d. Reevaluate your time again to see if you are going too fast.
6. Just slow down. Be methodical in reading and thinking.
7. Give yourself permission to be different next time, perhaps taking the entire time to complete the test.
8. Practice stopping just to put your mind at rest or on idle while focusing on your surroundings for 1 to 2 minutes. Do this at least twice a day.
   a. For example, when you find yourself waiting at a familiar stoplight, stop your thoughts. Look at the intersection and notice something new. Do this little exercise every time you are stopped by the red light at this intersection.

"Learn to pause . . . or nothing worthwhile will catch up to you."
Doug King

b. Exercises such as this challenge your thinking processes to look at common, familiar items in a different light. This will be helpful on tests when you encounter familiar words that, like the traffic signal, are cues to make a snap decision. You'll find you can simply redirect your attention to other words on the test item and form a more objective approach to the answer.

9. Focus on the content of test items and only the words that are written.

   a. It might be helpful to use a report approach, especially with questions that have multiple diagnoses and findings. To do this:

      i. Read the stem, questions, and options.

      ii. On your scrap paper, make notes of what you think is important. These notes should be like those that you take when getting reports from the prior shift. Put the data in order of priority as you write.

      iii. Be sure to use the abbreviations that you are familiar with. This helps you process the given data in a more objective manner.

      iv. Go back to the stem and reread the given data to see:

        (a) If you have missed important information.

        (b) If you have missed the priority concern.

        (c) If you added information or assumptions that were not actually stated.

      v. Read the question one more time.

      vi. Review your notes.

      vii. Read the options to narrow them to two or to make a final choice.

      viii. Repeat the process above until you have decided on a best option.

   b. Draw a picture of the situation or event.

10. Avoid false rules, such as "never clamp a chest

tube" or "always check vital signs first." These absolute rules lead to a tendency for subjectivity and insertion of extraneous information.

THE DECELERATOR

Directions: Check all that apply to you. During a test do you:

☐ Move slowly, methodically, and deliberately?

☐ Read, reread, and again reread?

☐ Reread with the insertion of information from your experiences or past knowledge of the given situation?

☐ End up consistently being the last one to finish the test?

☐ Have to rush to finish the last five to 10 items on the test?

☐ Read, think, and decide too slowly for each question?

☐ Have trouble deciding on most answers?

☐ Keep second-guessing yourself?

If you checked two or more of the above questions, you are a *decelerator.* You have a heavy foot on the brake and apply it frequently or forget to release the parking brake. You need to:

1. Put your watch in front of you during a test.
   a. Check the time after every 30 questions to see that you have not used more than 40 minutes.
   b. If you have used more than 40 minutes, speed up your pace for the next 30 questions to use no more than 35 minutes.
2. If taking a paper-pencil test, do not skip questions with the idea of going back to answer them at a later time.
3. Note the types of questions on which you spend more time. Are they associated with a specific issue, such as the following:
   a. Assessment?

b. Analysis?

    c. Intervention?

    d. Evaluation?

    e. A specific body system?

    f. A specific physiologic concept?

    g. Lab values?

4. Return to your reference book to read about any problem areas.

5. Once you identify problem areas, make up a story, metaphor, or image that helps you remember.

6. Every day do five questions, one at a time.

    a. Get out your timer, set it for 1 minute, then do one question.

    b. Note how much time you have left (the goal is 15 to 30 seconds). Keep in mind, however, that questions with long stems or long options will take longer than 30 to 45 seconds to complete.

7. Practice test questions. Do you go slower at the beginning of the test? Do you slow down in the middle, when a few of the previous questions have caused you to doubt your knowledge? Or do you go slower at the end, because you feel exhausted?

8. Use different approaches to reading the stem and the options.

    a. Most decelerators start with the first sentence and continue on in a methodical manner to end with option *d*.

    b. Many times, by the last option, decelerators have forgotten what the question is (just as they might forget that the emergency brake is on). By the time they have read option *d* they have a tendency to come up with a question to fit their answer.

        i. If the stem has a few sentences before the question, read the question first.

        ii. Next read the options from *a* to *d,* attempting to narrow the options to two out of the four.

        iii. Then read the information in the stem to identify whether any information is critical to make your selection of the best option.

iv. Upon selecting an option, do one last read of the question followed with the option you selected. If these make sense together, and if you haven't identified any missed key words, select that option as your answer and go on to the next question.

9. Eat before a test. An episode of hypoglycemia can hamper your ability to make simple decisions.

THE COASTER

Directions: Check all that apply to you. During a test do you:

☐ Rely largely on your personal experience with clients to help you select the best option?

☐ Have a tendency to think, "*My* information may not be the norm, the standard, or the expected, but it is *my* best guide to use on this question"?

☐ Have a tendency to focus on the one bit of information in the stem that you are most comfortable with and pay little attention to other details or data that are given?

☐ Select one option over another because it is what you did, or have seen, or have heard of being done in your hospital?

☐ Select an option because it most closely aligns with your hospital's policy or with familiar steps in a procedure?

If you checked two or more of the above questions, you are a *coaster* test-taker. You refuse to come to a complete stop, and instead coast by stop signs and through intersections. You say to your self, "This is about *me*; I go first at four-way stop signs!" You need to:

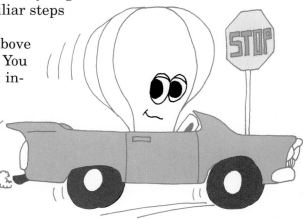

1. Focus on broad principles and standards that guide nursing actions.

Correct your course. You can't control the questions any more than a balloonist can control the wind! Accept what's actually on the page (or screen) and get back on course.

2. Think about priority questions in terms of the sequence:
   a. The ABCS (airway, breathing, and circulation—physiologic needs—and safety)
   b. Factors such as the following:
      i. Age
      ii. Developmental milestones
      iii. Environment
      iv. Education
      v. Time frames
3. Identify when you digress into the thinking patterns of "how we do it at our hospital." When this happens:
   a. Stop and close your eyes.
   b. Take three diaphragmatic breaths.
   c. Open your eyes and reread the question and options with a fresh mind.
4. Control your digressive behavior by one of the following actions:
   a. Close your eyes and take three slow, deep breaths, thinking or saying to yourself, "I will read the question and select my answer based on the given information."
   b. Close your eyes and take a mental mini-vacation to a relaxing, fun place. Return to the question and options with a renewed sense of observation.
   c. Close your eyes and think of nothing as you count from 1 to 10. Concentrate on picturing each digit on the inside of your eyelids as you count.

THE MUFFLER

Directions: Check all that apply to you. During a test do you:
   ☐ View tests as hurdles to jump?
   ☐ View tests as barriers to cross?
   ☐ View tests as threats to graduation?

☐ View tests as threats to your self-esteem ("If I fail, I'll just die"; or "If I fail, I'm stupid")?

☐ Find yourself preoccupied with grades?

☐ Face an upcoming test with the attitude of "I'll worry about it tomorrow"?

☐ Spend excess time and mental energy in avoidance of studying for the exam, rather than simply preparing for the test?

☐ Make excuses, valid or not, for your lack of preparation for the test?

If you checked two or more of the above questions, you are a *muffler*. You are like a car muffler that reduces noise—you tend to reduce all events to a fear or anxiety, whether appropriate or not. You need to:

1. Set a specific plan for progressive, disciplined study.
   a. Every day, spend 15 minutes reading over the notes from each class that day, making sure to do the following:
      i. Set your timer and reward yourself, then move on to the next set of class notes.
      ii. Read the major and minor headings in the chapter.
      iii. Identify areas that you need to study; take the time to read under that specific heading.
      iv. If you don't have the time to read in those areas, write the topic and page numbers you want to come back to on an index card.
         (1) Put this on your schedule to do during your next specified study time.
         (2) Or carry the book and index card with you to read during any 10 to 15 minutes of down time you might have (for example, between classes the next day, or while waiting for a family member

"What the mind can conceive and believe, the mind can achieve."
Napoleon Hill

after school). Use the index card with the page numbers as a bookmark.

    v. Remember, you sometimes don't have to read every word to develop an understanding of the material.

2. Incorporate defined, consistent time frames for completion into your unit review. Examples of this include the following:

    a. Take the unit in small bites; remember that test preparation is like eating an apple: a bite at a time gets the job done. So start out small. Tell yourself, "I'll sit down for 10 minutes to read over my notes every morning or every night." Set your timer, read, and stop when the timer goes off.

    b. Review in a new place. You may even try relating the choice of place to the organ or disease being studied. I associate the kitchen with the functions of the liver. In both, many processes take place that are vital to survival (in the kitchen, activities for the family; and in the liver, processes for the body).

3. Reward yourself often! Change your usual reward.

    a. Use time as a reward instead of other common self-rewards such as eating a favorite food, going shopping, or watching television.

        i. If you have spent 15 minutes reviewing notes, take 5 to 10 minutes to sit and do nothing, to read a few pages in a novel, or to talk to a friend.

        ii. Use caution! Keep a timer on your reward activity since you can easily get off track.

        iii. Get back to the task of test preparation for another short period after enjoying your reward of time.

4. Substitute a physical action for the use of mental energy in avoidance of exam preparation. This means to "do rather than dread." Be strict with yourself:

a. When you are thinking of doing other things instead of studying, force yourself to sit in a chair with your notes or book.

b. Open the book up!

c. Turn to a page of information you need to know.

d. Read the first page or paragraph.

e. This should get you jump-started to the first step in test preparation.

5. Avoid "grading" behaviors or answers such as the following:

a. "What a stupid action."

b. "The open-ended question is the best, no matter what."

THE SUNDAY DRIVER

Directions: Check all that apply to you. During a test do you:

☐ First, answer the question in the role of a student?

☐ Second, answer the question in the role of the teacher (for example, look to see if there is a "catch" or "trick" in the question or options)?

☐ Change your initial answer. Even change answers two to three times on one question?

☐ In options that have a series of items, do you make an initial choice based on knowledge, then change your choice when you reread the options based on one rather than all of the items in a series?

If you checked two or more of the above questions, you are a *Sunday driver.* You have a need to check out the route not just once, but many times; then you try six different ways to get to the same destination. You need to:

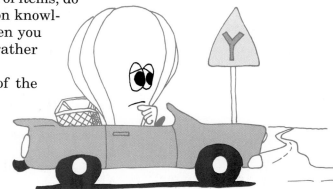

Create a map for yourself. Have an idea of what you are looking for.

1. Look at your pattern of changing answers.
   a. If changing answers more often results in the correct answer, keep changing.
2. If most of the time the initial selection is the correct answer, don't change your initial answer no matter what!
   a. How *not* to change answers:
      i. On a paper-pencil test, simply don't go back to any question. Answer each question as you go. This is also good practice for future tests that will be taken on a computer, since you usually can't go backwards on a computer exam.
      ii. On computer exams, reread only the options that you are unsure of or the two you have narrowed it down to. Do not reread all the options all the time!
      iii. Sit on your hands, especially at the beginning or end of the test when you are most likely to be tense or tired. This is a great reminder not to change your answers!
3. Move through the exam progressively and carefully.
   a. If you get stuck on two options (such as *a* and *c*), try reading them backwards.
      i. Read the question, then option *c*. Read the question, then option a, rather than reading in the more familiar sequence of the question, option *a*, and then option *c*.
      ii. Go with what you know! Don't second-guess. Have confidence in your perceptions and decisions.

THE DISTRACTED DRIVER

Directions: Check all that apply to you. During a test do you:

☐ Have an ability or tendency to formulate questions to get the most valuable informational response?

☐ Try to create the whole picture of the "who, what, where, why, when, and how" rather than the actual pieces of information given?

☐ Often veer away from selecting appropriate nursing responses because you've placed words or ideas that were really not intended into the statements?

☐ Have a tendency to reword the question or option to meet your train of thought?

☐ Read "between the lines" of statements given by clients?

☐ Have some tendency to separate emotions from actions?

If you checked two or more of the above questions you are a *distracted driver*. You have many stops and many excuses. You need to do the following:

1. Focus on the client.
2. Hear the client's thoughts and feelings as given in the stem or options.
3. Avoid formulating responses targeted at getting information.
4. Reflect on the client's remarks and perceptions of the situation or event.
5. Realize that you don't need all the information all the time.

Avoid being an "Info-holic" and letting analysis overwhelm your actions. Not all information is essential.

SUMMARY

Every test-taker has a different approach to testing, and these different approaches can be likened to the different types of drivers of vehicles. These characteristics may change over time. Therefore, it is a wise decision to re-evaluate your thoughts and actions every few quarters.

As with all habits, good and bad, we are typically

unaware of our actions unless we take the time to stop and review our behaviors. Specific prescriptions are effective for these various types of test-takers: speedsters, decelerators, coasters, mufflers, Sunday drivers, and distracted drivers. Look at life differently; try a new route.

The following poem or blessing is commonly heard after a balloon flight; it is my wish for you with *every* test life sends your way:

The Balloonists' Prayer

The winds have welcomed you with softness.
The sun has blessed you with his warm hands.
You have flown so high and so well
that God joined you in laughter
and set you gently back into
the loving arms of Mother Earth.

Author Unknown

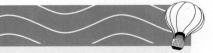

Air Currents

"Life, like a car, is driven from the inside out, not the other way around."

Richard Carlson

"The road to success starts when you are inspired to make an effort."

W. Clement Stone

Psychosynthesis: Be a Star Test-Taker

Patricia Romick

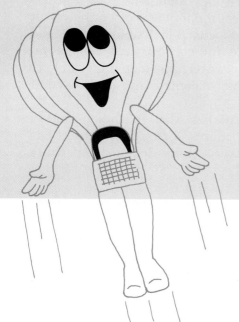

"Awareness is the essential ingredient in any process of growth. Without awareness, we can act only out of conditioning and habit."

Molly Young Brown

I really did not understand the art and skill of test-taking until 4 years ago.

Throughout my schooling, my test grades did not reflect my knowledge. My grades made me feel ashamed and inferior. Today, I know that my struggle with multiple choice exams was unnecessary, had there only been someone to teach me how to approach this type of test question.

A lack of focus will lead to a lack of confidence and control.

You may be wondering what happened 4 years ago to change this. I took a position as an academic and personal counselor to university nursing students. As a psychiatric/mental health clinical nurse specialist, I was experienced in personal counseling and realized that I had a learning curve to conquer regarding academic counseling, which includes test-taking skills.

The students with whom I worked helped me to understand why they chose the wrong answers on test questions, and I am indebted to them. It was from this information and observation that I began to understand that most multiple-choice questions are not missed because students have a content or knowledge deficit, but rather because students are unclear as to what they are being asked and what the answer options are suggesting.

I also noted that test anxiety was often the result of the student's lack of focus. A lack of focus will lead to a lack of confidence and control. Just as it is impossible to mix oil and water, it is also impossible to be anxious or to feel out of control and be focused at the same time.

This chapter explains the methods that I have used to help students focus. These methods depend on the ability to make decisions in three areas:

1. *What content* and *what about the content* (something just as important as the actual content) is being asked? Refer to the "focus technique" that follows.
2. How do the answer options relate to or distract from the content being tested? Refer to "push the pause button" later in this chapter.
3. How is freedom from test anxiety (tension or fatigue during the actual test) gained or achieved? Refer to "the star model for success in testing" later in this chapter.

FOCUS TECHNIQUE

Step One

As you read the test question, underline the words in each question that answer *what content* and *what about the content* is being asked. Underline individual key words as you read. This is not an exercise in underlining; it is an exercise in *thinking* as you underline. For example, if your content is pneumonia, you begin to think "lungs, respiratory, and infection." If your *what about* the content is "manifestation of pneumonia," you begin to think "cough, fever, and lethargy." Do this process regardless of the length of the question; no question is too short for this process.

Age, sex, diagnosis, clinical manifestations, lab values, and vital signs are all significant items to be underlined. Also underline *who* is being asked about, the *nurse,* the *client,* or the *family?* Be aware of words such as *most, best, except, first, primary, acute, chronic,* and other adjectives. Be alert to phrases such as *"is scheduled for," "upon completion of the admission," "as the condition improves,"* or *"in preparation for discharge."* These give you the time parameters for the given situation.

When you underline, do not use a continuous line; underline individual words one at a time. Each word underlined needs to "pop out" at you so that those words will then direct you to the best option. Try out this underlining technique on the following questions:

> *Ask yourself:* <u>What</u> <u>content</u> and <u>what</u> <u>about</u> <u>the</u> <u>content</u> is being asked?

> *Underline each key word individually to make the word "pop out" at you.*

1. A client is scheduled for a colonoscopy. The most serious complication associated with this procedure is:
   a. Constipation
   b. Severe abdominal cramping
   c. Infection following the procedure
   d. Perforation of the bowel

2. The most valuable therapeutic communication technique to be used during the assessment of the psychosocial domain in the elderly client is:
   a. Listening
   b. Touching
   c. Smiling
   d. Nodding
3. The immobilized client is prone to the development of hypostatic pneumonia. To prevent this, the nurse would:
   a. Encourage hyperventilation
   b. Order prophylactic antibiotics
   c. Assist the client to turn, cough, and breathe deeply
   d. Teach the client about the dangers of overexertion and encourage rest

Do your decisions match mine? Here they are:

1. A client is scheduled for a <u>colonoscopy.</u> The <u>most serious complication</u> associated with this procedure is:
   a. Constipation
   b. Severe abdominal cramping
   c. Infection following the procedure
   d. Perforation of the bowel

   The *content* in this question is "colonoscopy"; *what about the content* is "most serious complication." The word "colonoscopy" directs you to the bowel; "most serious" directs you to perforation.

2. The <u>most</u> <u>valuable</u> <u>therapeutic communication technique</u> to be used during the <u>assessment</u> of the <u>psychosocial domain</u> in the elderly client is:
   a. Listening
   b. Touching
   c. Smiling
   d. Nodding

The *content* of this question is "assessment of the psychosocial domain of the elderly" and the *what about the content* is "most valuable therapeutic communication technique." The word "assessment" directs you to listening or touching. So smiling and nodding would be the first two options eliminated. "Most valuable" and "assessment of the psychosocial domain" direct you to listening, option *a*.

3. The <u>immobilized</u> client is <u>prone</u> <u>to</u> the <u>development</u> of <u>hypostatic</u> <u>pneumonia</u>. <u>To</u> <u>prevent</u> this, the <u>nurse</u> <u>would</u>:
   a. Encourage hyperventilation
   b. Order prophylactic antibiotics
   c. Assist the client to turn, cough, and breathe deeply
   d. Teach the client about the dangers of overexertion and encourage rest

The *content* is "immobilized client." The *what about the content* is "to prevent hypostatic pneumonia." The word "immobilized" reflects the need for movement, eliminating *d* as an option, and directs you to turn, cough, and breathe deeply, option c. The word "nurse" in the stem eliminates *b* as an option.

Step Two

As you read the options, eliminate the two that could not be right as a result of your content knowledge. Read each word in every option because part of the option could be right and part of it could be wrong! *Never* choose an option without reading *all* of the options or all of the parts of one option.

Take the two remaining options individually back to your underlined words in the question to determine the best option. Most of the time there is a clear hint in those words "popping out" at you, as you will note in the following examples:

Never choose an option before reading every word of all the options!

1. Which of the following <u>contains</u> <u>all</u> the <u>elements</u> necessary for <u>informed</u> <u>consent?</u>
   a. The nurse explains the operative procedure and obtains the client's written consent.
   b. Any hospital employee may obtain the client's signature on the consent form.
   c. The physician explains the operative procedure and obtains the client's consent on a form that specifically identifies the procedure.
   d. The client signs the consent for the specified procedure after the physician explains the procedure and associated risks.

   The key words popping out are "all elements" and "informed consent." In options *a* and *b*, the words "written consent" and "consent form" are different from "informed consent," so they are eliminated first. Let's take a look at options *c* and *d* and compare them to the key words "all elements." We note that option *d* adds "associated risks," which is an element missing from option *c*. Option *c* only addresses the "procedure." Option *d* is more comprehensive. Therefore, option *d* is the best and correct option.

2. <u>Diabetes mellitus</u> is the <u>most</u> <u>common</u> <u>disorder</u> of <u>glucose</u> <u>regulation</u> <u>owing</u> <u>to</u> a <u>decreased</u> amount or <u>absence</u> of <u>insulin</u> that <u>results</u> <u>in</u> <u>abnormal</u> <u>metabolism</u> <u>of:</u>
   a. Carbohydrates
   b. Protein
   c. Fat
   d. Carbohydrates, protein, and fat

   In this question, the key words "diabetes mellitus" and "abnormal metabolism" direct us to *a* and *d* as possibilities because they have carbohydrates as part of the answer. Options *b* and *c* are eliminated first. Thus if protein and fat are wrong in options *b* and *c*, they are wrong in option *d*, leaving option *a* as the correct option.

PUSH THE PAUSE BUTTON

When you do not know the correct option and are going to guess, try the following five actions:

1. Don't panic! Pause, take three slow, deep breaths; then use your common sense, critical thinking skills, and reading comprehension skills.
2. Do not read *into* the question. Only think about the words presented to you in the questions and the options. If you add words to either (in your thinking), you have lost your focus. Write a few notes on your paper about what you *think* you are reading, then compare these to the words on the computer screen.
3. Be cautious in choosing an option that has "absolute" words in it or that is phrased in an absolute manner. In addition to *all* and *none,* other absolutes are *completely, totally, always, forever, an absence of,* and *never.*
4. Remember, *content* cannot be in the *option* if it is not in the *question or stem.* For example, if the content is about the kidneys or bladder, and two of the options relate to the brain or the musculoskeletal system, those options would be eliminated first.
5. Look at your options and find two that are similar but dissimilar. Try this example:

When the diagnosis of diabetes was confirmed, the client became very upset. This emotional <u>stress</u> would typically <u>cause:</u>

    a. A decrease in blood sugar
    b. An increase in blood sugar
    c. No change in blood sugar
    d. A decrease in medication

Notice that options *a* and *b* are similar with one exception: decrease versus increase. So if I'm going to guess at one of the above answers, I'm going to guess between options *a* or *b.* The correct answer is option *b.*

Push the pause button when you don't know the correct option and are about to guess.

Try another example:

The nurse takes the <u>blood pressure</u> of an <u>obese</u> client. If the nurse uses a <u>standard-sized</u> blood pressure <u>cuff,</u> the <u>blood pressure reading</u> may be:

a. Falsely low
b. Falsely high
c. Indistinct
d. More time consuming

Again note that options *a* and *b* are similar with one exception: low versus high. If I'm going to guess, I'm going to guess at one of those two options. The correct answer is option *b*.

Here is a different kind of example for guessing at options that are similar but dissimilar:

A 145-lb., active, 91-year-old man falls while painting his garage. He is admitted to your unit with a <u>fractured hip.</u> He does not like hospital food and refuses to eat. This client's <u>basic caloric need during hospitalization</u> is expected to:

a. Decrease because of his inactivity
b. Decrease because of his advanced age
c. Increase because of his normally high activity level
d. Increase because of his fracture

As a skilled test-taker, the first thing you have to do in this kind of question is to decide which pair of similar, but dissimilar options are to be focused on. The *content* here is a client with an "acute fractured hip"; the *what about the content* is "expected basic caloric need during hospitalization." So, you think "fractured hip means injury, which will need to heal, so this requires an increase in calories." The decision is to eliminate options *a* and *b* and focus on options *c* or *d*. Note that in option *c* new information is introduced into the situation—a "high" activity level. In the stem the client is described as an "active" 91-year-old man. In contrast, option *d* refers back to the "fracture." The best option is *d*.

At this point, you may be saying to yourself,

"Well, this is all fine if I'm dealing with a paper test where I will be able to underline the *content*. But this will be useless if it is a computer test." Don't be hasty in jumping to that conclusion. After practicing on paper, the important words will automatically "pop out" at you on a computer. You have already established the habit of focusing and being clear as to what the words in questions and options are saying to you!

PSYCHOSYNTHESIS AND TEST-TAKING

The discussion of test-taking tips in the first part of this chapter applies principles of psychosynthesis. *Psychosynthesis* is a holistic view of health. It recognizes that what affects one part of us affects all other parts: body, mind, and spirit. It is a flexible set of tools and methods that aim at integrating the many parts that make up who we are, the strength, skill, and goodness of our *will,* and our inner wisdom. It is a psychological theory and method for describing and working with our personalities.

Psychosynthesis can be applied to testing situations to improve performance. The remainder of this chapter shows you how to apply some of these principles and tools of psychosynthesis to test-taking and academic success in nursing. My star model of academic student success was inspired by psychosynthesis founder Dr. R. Assagioli, who developed the star image of the personality.

> *Psychosynthesis is a holistic view of health that integrates who we are, our self, and our will.*

THE STAR MODEL FOR SUCCESS IN TESTING

As you soar toward success in test-taking, remember to reach toward the stars and find your unique star, the one that illustrates who you are with all of your qualities and skills to be academically successful. Let's discuss the star model (Figure 12-1).

The *self* at the center of the star represents your awareness of identity, centeredness, and individuality. *Centeredness* is your point of balance and integration. Relaxation responses, imagery, and affirmations—all tools of psychosynthesis—can be used to

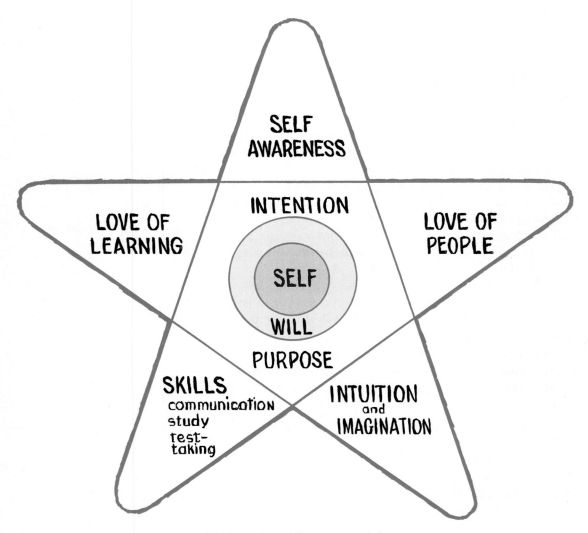

Figure 12-1 The star model.

direct your focus inward and find the quiet place within where your true, centered self resides. This is your place of pure self-awareness and knowing, the place where you can use mental actions to select the better of two answer options during a test.

Box 12-1 provides a psychosynthesis imagery exercise that will assist you in finding your place of self-awareness and centeredness. I suggest that you tape this exercise in your own voice and allow the tape to guide you whenever you feel the need.

Next, as you can see in the star model, the *will* is placed close to the *self*. That is because, according to Dr. Assagioli, we are willful beings and our will houses our skill, strength, and goodness. The self directs these aspects of the will. If you clarify your intent to do well on a test and align your intent with the skill, strength, and goodness of your will, you greatly enhance the probability that you will achieve your purpose or goal of success on the test. The will and the self continuously interact. The phases of the will in action are compared to the steps of the nursing process in Table 12-1.

In addition to the self-awareness that comes from self-identification and will identification, your academic success can be enhanced if you have or develop a love for learning. You can change the learning process into an adventure if you incorporate your attitudes, values, feelings, intuition, and imagination into your educational experience. Without the use of these aspects of learning and knowing, your mind is only used in assimilating content. Assimilation of content into the mind is less exciting, less stimulating, and at times just plain boring.

You may have noticed, as you explored objective test-taking skills earlier in this chapter, that getting to the best option requires not only your thinking mind, but also your intuition and imagination. Intuition and imagination arise from the unconscious mind. The material you learn for tests can be found both in your conscious awareness and your uncon-

Clarify your intent to do well on a test and align your intent with the skill, strength, and goodness of your will. Doing so will help you achieve your purpose or goal of success.

Change the learning process into an adventure by incorporating your attitudes, values, feelings, intuition, and imagination into your educational experience.

Box 12-1

Self-Identification Exercise

Begin by using a relaxation method that is familiar to you. If you do not have one, then try this one.

Sit in a comfortable position with your feet on the floor. Take several deep breaths and begin to allow your body to relax. Notice the places in your body that stop your breath from moving fully to the top of your head with each inhalation and to the bottom of your feet with each exhalation. Simply notice this without judgment, and continue to breathe normally, allowing each breath to continue to relax your body. Then listen to the following affirmations which you have recorded on an audiotape:

I have a body but I am not my body. My body is sometimes healthy, sick, rested, or tired, but my body is not who *I* am. I value my body as a tool of experience and action in the world. I attempt to treat it well and pursue efforts to keep it healthy, but my body is not my *self*. I have a body but I am not my body.

I have emotions but I am not my emotions. My emotions change sometimes from moment to moment, hour to hour, day to day. My emotions sway from love to hate, calm to anger, joy to grief, and yet my true *self* does not change. I remain. Although a ripple of emotion may at the moment immerse me, it will pass with time; thus I am not this emotion. I have emotions but I am not my emotions.

I have desires but I am not my desires. Desires are intensified by physical and emotional drives and frequently change and contradict one another. I have desires but I am not my desires.

I have a mind but I am not my mind. I value my mind for its capacity to think, learn, communicate, and experience, but my mind is not who *I* am. Often, my mind refuses to obey me; thus it can not be my *self*. I have a mind but I am not my mind.

I have many roles in life, but I am not my roles. My role may be that of son or father; daughter or mother; wife, husband, or significant other; student or teacher. But *I* am more than any role. I have many roles but I am not any of them. I have roles but I am not my roles.

Who am *I* then if I am not my body, my emotions and feelings, my desires, my mind and thoughts, or my roles? What am *I* then? *I* am a living, loving, willing being. *I* am a center of pure self-identity, awareness, and consciousness. *I* am more than the sum of the parts of who I am.

I recognize and affirm myself as a living, loving, willing being. *I* recognize and affirm that I am a center of pure self-awareness and creative self-expression. I understand that from this center of true identity I can observe, direct, and integrate my body, mind, and spirit.

Adapted from the original Identification Exercise developed by Roberto Assagioli, MD.

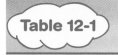 **Table 12-1**

The Phases of the Will in Action Compared to the Steps in the Nursing Process

Nursing Process Steps	The Will in Action	Application to Test-Taking
Assessing	Purpose-aim-goal–based evaluation, motivation, and intention	Goal: academic success based on self-assessment of nursing knowledge and test-taking skill, intention, and motivation.
Diagnosing	Deliberation	What grade do I want? Am I willing to do what it takes? What content do I need to study? Do I need tutoring? Am I being an effective time-manager? What is going on in my life that *detracts* and what is going on that *benefits* the attention I can give to test preparation?
Planning	Choice and decision empowerment	Do I choose to do what it takes? Do I choose to prepare for tests in the following manner? <ul><li>Prepare for each class by reading assignment before class.</li><li>Write out objectives in each chapter (write enough to understand content and application of content).</li><li>Write out glossary terms in each assigned chapter.</li><li>Take complete notes in class.</li><li>Come to class with questions.</li><li>Study class handouts.</li><li>Prior to test, review all of the above.</li></ul>

Continued

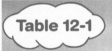

Table 12-1 | **The Phases of the Will in Action Compared to the Steps in the Nursing Process—cont'd**

Nursing Process Steps	The Will in Action	Application to Test-Taking
Implementing	Affirmation planning and working out a program	Affirm yourself by completing the statements in Box 12-2.
		Use relaxation and affirmation self-imagery to create a relaxed confidence in your ability to succeed. Make your own tape as a guide to focus these thoughts. (See the sample script in Box 12-3.)
		Write out your plan for your program success with specific plans for studying and learning.
		Use time-management skills of keeping written "daily things to do lists"; and weekly, monthly, and quarterly calendars showing class and clinical times, study times, scheduled tests with deadlines for study times, written assignment schedules, rest and recreation times, and other social, home, or work commitments.
Evaluating	Direction of the progress	Reconnect with your purpose of obtaining a nursing degree and becoming a licensed professional nurse.
	Execution to include mental and physical action	Clarify your intention to be successful.
		Align your intent with the skill, strength, and goodness of your will.
	Supervision and evaluation	Evaluate your progress and course of preparation: Am I on target? If not, how did I miss it and what were the pitfalls?

> **Box 12-2**

Affirmation for Test-Takers

I have now made a grade of _____ on my test.

I see _____.
I hear _____.
I feel _____.
I smell _____.
I touch _____.
I sense _____.

This has now happened for me. Thank you.

SAMPLE AFFIRMATION

I have now made a "B" on my pharmacology test.

   I *see* the grade on my e-mail.

   I *hear* my best friend congratulating me on my grade.

   I *feel* that my grade reflects the amount of time and effort I felt I could devote to test preparation.

   I *smell* the salt from the ocean in the air as I drive to school to get my grade.

   I *touch* my friends as they hug me in support.

   I *sense* joy as I learn of my grade.

   This has now happened for me. Thank you.

   Note: Affirmations are written as if they have already happened. Affirmations are a result of having made a choice and utilizing the *will* in action. The *skillful will* in action collects your thoughts, emotions, sensations, and desires regarding your choice. Your *strong will* provides the strength to carry out your choice. Your *good will* ensures that the choice is not harmful to you or others.

scious mind. This is why your first hunch about the right option on a test question is often correct.

   Attitudes, feelings, and values related to the love of people can have a large influence on your commitment to learning and on the successful demonstration of your competencies as a nursing student.

Attitudes, feelings, and values related to the love of people can have a large influence on your success as a nursing student.

Box 12-3

Relaxation Exercise for the Star Test-Taker

Record the following script on an audiotape. Then sit in a comfortable chair and play back the audiotape. (You may want to record a tape for a friend.)

Allow yourself to close your eyes and rest both feet on the ground. Take several deep breaths, allowing the air to move up through your body with each inhalation and down through your body with each exhalation. (Pause.) Resume your natural pattern of breathing. Remember, breathing is effortless, so just allow it to happen. (Pause.) Notice how your breath begins to relax your body; each breath relaxes your body more and more. As your breath continues to relax your body, also let it relax your mind. Let go of any thoughts or feelings that are on your mind. (Pause.) Let each breath, as it continues to relax your body, clear your mind of thoughts and feelings, relaxing your mind. (Pause.) Begin to notice, with your body and mind relaxed, the quiet place deep within you that is self-aware and centered. (Pause.) This is your place of knowing; this is your place of awareness. (Pause.) From this place of knowing, imagine yourself doing extremely well on the test you are about to take. (Pause.) See or sense yourself feeling centered and confident. See or sense yourself staying calm and focused as you go from question to question, from answer option to answer option. See or sense yourself reading each question and answer option completely. See or sense yourself discovering the clues that lead you to the correct option. See or sense yourself marking the correct option. See or sense yourself filled with excitement and joy as you discover how well you have done on this test. See or sense yourself rejoicing with your family and friends over your test success. (Pause.) Be aware that you can access this place of knowing within you at any time simply by using your imagination to return to it. Now allow your awareness to return to the room, noticing your body sitting on the chair, noticing your thoughts and feelings, and opening your eyes.

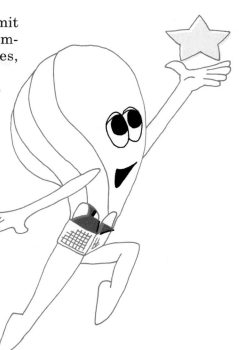

- If you value communication, you will commit to learning how to become a therapeutic communicator with your clients, their families, and your team members.
- If you value human life, you will commit to doing whatever it takes to become a competent, safe practitioner.
- If you respect the dignity of the individual, you will commit to learning about acceptance and tolerance of individual differences among your clients.
- Loving people also means loving yourself. It is impossible to love others without first loving yourself.

SUMMARY

You can become a star test-taker by these simple actions anchored in psychosynthesis:

1. Knowing and understanding yourself through self-awareness and self-identification.
2. Recognizing your inner strength and wisdom as characterized in the aspects of your will: strength, skill, and goodness.
3. Using effective communication, study, and test-taking skills.
4. Using your intuition and imagination as well as your thinking, conscious mind.
5. Becoming passionate about your love for learning and for people.
6. Connecting with your purpose and clarifying your intentions.

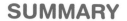

Soar toward success in test-taking by finding your star, the one that illustrates who you are with all of your qualities and skills.

It is important to be aware of your thoughts about studying and learning; it is also essential to have an awareness of your feelings about the components of successful test-taking.

Stay aware of:

Recognize your thoughts and feelings about learning.

- How you feel about wanting to learn.
- How you feel as you are learning.
- How you feel after you have learned.

Recognize your *thoughts* and *feelings* about learning so that you can:

- Assess
- Analyze
- Plan
- Implement
- Evaluate your test preparation needs

Combining the application of psychosynthesis and the nursing process can enhance your motivation, empowerment, and self-esteem as you soar toward becoming a star test-taker.

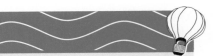

Air Currents

"I shall suggest a few phrases, taken from inscriptions on the coats of arms of various noble families:

   Ad sidera vultus—*Face toward the stars*
   Pensa al fine—*Think of the goal*
   Bien faire et laisser dire—*Act well and
     let people talk*
   Semper vigilans—*Ever watchful*
   In tutto armonia—*In everything,
     harmony"*

Roberto Assagioli

"Let us run with perseverance the race that is set before us."

Hebrews 12:1

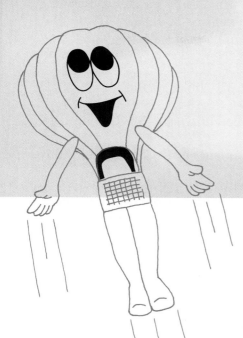

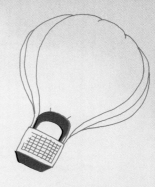

Bibliography

CHAPTERS 1-11

Aslett D: *How to have a 48-hour day,* Pocatello, Idaho, 1996, Marsh Creek Press.

Ban Breathnach S: *Simple abundance journal of gratitude,* New York, N.Y., 1996, Warner Books.

Blair L: *Passport to practical and vocational nursing,* St. Louis, 1998, Mosby.

Carlson R: *Don't sweat the small stuff . . . and it's all small stuff,* New York, N.Y., 1997, Hyperion Press.

Grainger RD: Managing fatigue, *Am J Nurs,* 90(3): 13, 1990.

Higgs LC: *Forty reasons why life is more fun after the big 40,* Nashville, 1997, Thomas Nelson Publishers.

Johnson B: *Living somewhere between estrogen and death,* Dallas, 1997, Word Publishing.

Kirchheimer S, Malesky G: *Energy forever,* Emmaus, Pa., 1997, Rodale Press.

Paul R: Paper prepared for the National Council for Excellence in Critical Thinking, Rohnert Park, Calif., 1993, Sonoma State University.

Peale NV: *Stay alive all your life,* Pawling, N.Y., 1957, Prentice-Hall, Inc.

Peale NV: *The power of positive thinking,* Pawling, N.Y., 1952, 1978, Prentice-Hall, Inc.

Peale NV: *How to handle a problem successfully, audiotape,* Pawling, N.Y., 1980, Foundation for Christian Living.

Rollant P: Acing multiple-choice questions, *AJN Career Guide for 1994,* 36:18-21, 1994.

Rollant P: *Mosby's review cards,* St. Louis, 1997, Mosby.

Rollant P: *Mosby's review series,* St. Louis, 1996, Mosby.

Rollant P: Success on the NCLEX-RN exam: try this tripod approach, *Nursing 92,* 22(10):6-13, 1992.

Sherman C: *Stress remedies,* Emmaus, Pa., 1997, Rodale Press.

Stone WC: *The success system that never fails,* Englewood Cliffs, N.J., 1962, Prentice-Hall, Inc.

Thompson C: *What a great idea,* New York, N.Y., 1992, Harper Perennial.

Von Oech R: *A whack to the side of the head,* Stamford, Conn., 1990, U.S. Games Sytems, Inc.

Von Oech R: *A kick in the seat of the pants,* New York, N.Y., 1986, Harper and Row.

Wycoff J: *Mindmapping: your personal guide to exploring creativity and problem-solving,* New York, N.Y., 1991, Berkley Books.

CHAPTER 12

Assagioli R: *The act of will,* New York, N.Y., 1973, Penguin.

Brown MY: *Growing whole,* New York, N.Y., 1993, HarperCollins.

Ferrucci P: *What we may be,* New York, N.Y., 1982, GP Putnam's Sons.

Montgomery CL: *Healing through communication: the practice of caring,* Newbury Park, Calif., 1993, Sage.

Romick P: Psychosynthesis: a perspective for growth and healing for self. In Kritek PB, editor: *Reflections on healing: a central nursing construct,* New York, N.Y., 1997, National League for Nursing Press.

Rowan J: *Subpersonalities: the people inside us,* London, 1990, Routledge.

Whitmore D: *Psychosynthesis in education,* Rochester, Vt., 1986, Destiny Books.

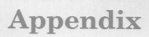

Appendix **A**

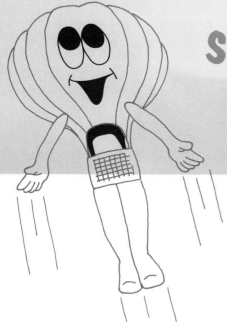

Self-Diagnostic Profile for Testing Errors

PROBLEM AREA IDENTIFICATION WITH PRESCRIPTIONS

Directions:

Step 1. After you complete a test of multiple choice questions, such as the test found in Appendix B, and as you are checking for the missed questions, review this list of common errors. Place one check mark in the errors column after the specific error *for each time the error occurred.*

Step 2. Note where your errors cluster. Eliminate these errors by using the prescriptions that follow.

Test-Taking Problem Area	Errors
I. Content or Concept	
• Unknown	
• Forgot	
• Unable to recall correct part	
• Applied incorrectly	
II. Critical Elements	
Missed:	
• Key words	
• Time elements	
• A step in the nursing process	
Assessment	
Analysis	
Planning	
Intervention	
Evaluation	
• Details such as *in*accurate	
• Knew answer, but selected incorrect answer	
• Had an emotional response to question	
• Thought question was stupid or inappropriate	
III. Questions	
• Misread	
• Read into	
• Drew wrong conclusion	
• Missed important point	
• Didn't read all of the question or stem	
• Incorrectly evaluated distractors	
• Chose wrong word as being important	
IV. Options	
• Misread	
• Read into	
• Drew wrong conclusion	
• Missed important point	
• Didn't read all options	
• Incorrectly evaluated distractors	
• Chose wrong word as being important	

Prescriptions

I. Content or Concept

During review of a test:

1. Keep a log of the content from any missed questions.
2. Once a week look up the content and associate it with something familiar and fun.
3. (Add your own.)

During a test:

1. Do one exercise each for mental and physical tension and tiredness reduction:
   a. Before doing questions
   b. Every 25 questions for tests <100 questions
   c. Every 50 questions for tests >100 questions
   d. When you get tired or tense
2. Reread the question with your selected option for validation of your choice of options as the last step before going to the next test question.
3. Read the options with just noun and verb.
   a. Attempt to apply a theme to the options, such as internal, external, or systems-focused.
4. (Add your own.)

II. Critical Elements

During the test:

1. Check for tenseness or fatigue routinely or when you are having difficulty. These feelings may decrease your perception and thinking skills.
   a. Check to see if you are doing practice questions during times of greater fatigue, such as after work.
   b. Reorganize your schedule to do practice questions when you are fresher.
   c. Do daily mental and/or physical stress reduction exercises so they become part of your daily routine, like brushing your teeth.

2. Read the question, then the options in a sequence from option *d* to option *a* instead of the traditional way of reading from option *a* to option *d*.
   a. Select an option.
   b. Reread the question with your selected option to validate your choice.
3. Use the cluster technique on the options.
   a. Group three options into a similar theme or category.
   b. The odd option out is most likely the best option to answer the question.
   c. Use this action only if you have no idea of a correct answer!

During review of the test answers that you got wrong:

1. Reread the stem, the question, and all the options.
2. Look for key words, time frames, or other elements that you may have overlooked or misread.

III. and IV. Questions and Options

1. Do a mental and physical tension reduction exercise before starting the exam and after every 25 questions during the exam.
2. Use the following *process of reading* on the more difficult questions or if you have narrowed the answer to two options:
   a. Read the question, followed by the information in the stem.
   b. Read the options and determine which two are the best.
   c. Identify key words or time frames that may have been missed:
      i. Reread the question with option 1.
      ii. Then reread the question with option 2.
   d. Select the best option.
   e. Do one last reread of the question with your selected option.

3. If you have a tendency not to read all of the options:
   a. Read the options in a sequence from option d to option a instead of the traditional way of option a through to option d.
   b. Do this method of reading on your practice tests first, since this change will often cause you some degree of tension, anxiety, or fatigue.

ERROR PATTERN IDENTIFICATION WITH PRESCRIPTIONS

Directions:

Step 1. Immediately after any exam, either practice or real, write down the number of test questions and any influencing factors that may have occurred before or during the test (such as a sick child, argument, accident, low or high energy, or any other causes of tension or fatigue).

Step 2. After you have corrected the test, determine where most of your wrong answers were grouped on the test (in relation to the beginning, middle, or end).

Exam 1

Pattern of incorrect questions in a _____ item exam.
Influencing factors:

- Missed more on the first third of exam
- Missed more on the middle of exam
- Missed more on the last third of exam
- No pattern noted

Exam 2

Pattern of incorrect questions in a _____ item exam.
Influencing factors:

- Missed more on the first third of exam
- Missed more on the middle of exam
- Missed more on the last third of exam
- No pattern noted

Exam 3

Pattern of incorrect questions in a _____ item exam.
Influencing factors:

- Missed more on the first third of exam
- Missed more on the middle of exam
- Missed more on the last third of exam
- No pattern noted

Exam 4

Pattern of incorrect questions in a _____ item exam.
Influencing factors:

- Missed more on the first third of exam
- Missed more on the middle of exam
- Missed more on the last third of exam
- No pattern noted

Exam 5

Pattern of incorrect questions in a _____ item exam.
Influencing factors:

- Missed more on the first third of exam
- Missed more on the middle of exam
- Missed more on the last third of exam
- No pattern noted

Summary of Your Pattern of Errors

Based on your pattern, where do you miss more questions? This is where you need to do tenseness and fatigue reduction exercises. Remember to do a physical and a mental exercise because combining them is more efficient and effective.

Pattern of incorrect questions in <100-item exam: select one of the items in the right column.	• Missed more on the first third of exam • Missed more on the middle of exam • Missed more on the last third of exam • No pattern noted
Pattern of incorrect questions in 100 to 200-item exam: select one of the items in the right column.	• Missed more on the first third of exam • Missed more on the middle of exam • Missed more on the last third of exam • No pattern noted
Pattern of incorrect questions in >200-item exam: select one of the items in the right column.	• Missed more on the first third of exam • Missed more on the middle of exam • Missed more on the last third of exam • No pattern noted

Prescriptions

1. Note where your pattern of errors occurred with the different lengths of exams.
2. If you can recall or if you kept a log of influencing factors for each test situation:
   a. Were you tired or tense at the section of the exam where you missed more questions?
   b. Were there any disruptions on the day of the exam?
      i. Physical illness of self or family members
      ii. Family crisis or problems
      iii. Work crisis or problems
      iv. Low energy
   c. Is there a pattern to the type of disruptions you have associated with testing?
      i. Are these within your control to change?
         (1) If yes, stop now. Think of one action to change this disruption.
         (2) Write it down now, here:

         (3) Write it on your calendar the week before your next practice or real exam to remind yourself to do this new behavior.
      ii. Are they out of your control?
         (1) If yes, stop now. Think of a way you can control your reaction (perhaps mentally shelve the problem).
         (2) Write it down now, here:

3. Do one mental and one physical exercise each at the beginning, middle, and end of that section where your pattern of errors occurred.
4. On tests with more than 100 questions, do mental and/or physical exercises after every 50 questions.

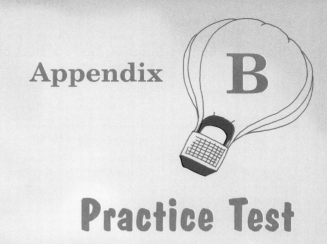

Appendix B

Practice Test

BEFORE THE TEST

During this test, what exercises will you use when you get tired or tense?

Physical

1.
2.

Mental

1.
2.

When or how often do you expect to use them?

Write down the name of a person who has faith in your abilities.

Now picture this person at your side lending support.

AFTER THE TEST

Review the questions that you have missed. Place each incorrect answer in one of the following two categories based on what caused you to select it. As you do this, write the category abbreviation (C or M) next to each incorrect answer.

1. Lacked content knowledge—C
2. Misread or misinterpreted the question—M

Identify where your major difficulty lies by filling in the chart on the following page.

On questions missed from a lack of content knowledge, go back to find where you could have:

- Made an association between the information and the option.
- Associated the organ involved with a step in the nursing process or a general physiologic or psychological concept.
- Identified an association among the options or between two options.

On questions missed as a result of misreading or misinterpretation, go back to find how you could have:

Type of Problem	Number of Incorrect Answers	Actions Needed to Remedy Problem
Lack of Content Knowledge		
Misread or Misinterpreted Question		

- Avoided reading into the questions or options.
- Identified key words or other clues (a step in the nursing process, the time frame, or an interaction between organs or body systems).
- Focused on "what about the content" was being asked in addition to "what content" was being tested.

With practice and repetition you will be able to select the best answer for any question.

QUESTIONS

1. An elderly client admitted to the hospital from a homeless shelter has these lab results returned: ALT, LDH, and AST elevated, WBC slightly elevated, minimal alcohol present, and BUN of 55. In addition to confusion and visual hallucinations, what other manifestations of delirium tremens does the nurse anticipate in this client?
   a. Hyper-jaundiced sclera
   b. Flapping tremors
   c. Irritability with little things
   d. Seizure activity

2. After radical neck surgery a client has two tubes leading from the incision site to a portable wound drainage system. The client reports an uncomfortable feeling of swelling in the neck area. The drainage system is checked and is patent for some serosanguineous drainage. The nurse should next evaluate for which of these anticipated findings?
   a. Loss of the gag reflex
   b. An increased level of consciousness
   c. Dehiscence of the suture line
   d. Severe difficulty in swallowing

3. The nurse assesses the interpersonal relations of an elderly client with a severe depressive disorder. Which of these questions should the nurse ask during the initial interview for admission to the unit?
   a. Do others criticize you?
   b. Do you feel isolated from others?
   c. Tell me about the degree of control in your life.
   d. Tell me about the past few days in your life.

4. An adolescent admitted for sickle cell anemia is to be discharged. The nurse reviews with the client the complications that can occur if the sickling process takes place. The adolescent indicates a readiness for the return home if, in a discussion of the reasons for sickling to occur, the client identifies which of these findings?
   a. Some loss of blood
   b. A temperature of 102
   c. Loss of strength on one side of the body
   d. Severe increase in thirst after a vigorous workout at the gym

5. A client at 36 weeks gestation reports an episode of exquisite abdominal pain. What assessment finding of this manifestation is most likely?
   a. Placenta previa
   b. Abruptio placentae
   c. A ruptured uterus
   d. A fetal incident

6. The nurse notes that a client's serum creatinine level is up to 5 from a level of 2 taken just 3 days ago. The nurse's first actions should be to:
   a. Call the lab to repeat the test and notify the physician.
   b. Check the client's neurologic state and labs for changes in serum potassium levels.
   c. Take the client's vital signs and ask for the ECG report from that morning.
   d. Check the client's level of consciousness and monitor the client's pulse for irregularities and rapidity.

7. Which of these findings reported by the mother of a 4-month-old infant suggest the onset of a higher than normal digoxin level in the infant?
   a. Nausea
   b. Listlessness
   c. Poor feeding
   d. A racing heart rate

8. What "best sequence" should the nurse teach the client for the use of beclomethasone dipropionate (Beclovent) in preparation for an acute asthma event?
   a. After the bronchodilator
   b. Before the bronchodilator
   c. Before respiratory treatments
   d. Upon the initial feeling of having an asthma attack

9. A client receives aminophylline for an acute exacerbation of bronchitis. The nurse is alert that the expected reportable effects of this drug are which of these manifestations?
   a. An increase in productivity and liquidity of pulmonary secretions
   b. A decrease in the frequency of coughing
   c. A sustained heart rate of 110 from a baseline of 60
   d. A feeling of nervousness with client reports of "twitching muscles"

10. A postmenopausal client talks with the nurse about vitamin B_{12} injectable. Which statement by the client reflects a need for the nurse to clarify information?
   a. "I can expect no change in the color of my stools."
   b. "I need to come to the office for bimonthly injections."

c. "I believe I will have more energy."

d. "The substance from the stomach is minimally available to absorb this vitamin if I take it by mouth."

11. A client on an oral anticoagulant should avoid selection of which food in the cafeteria line?
   a. Cabbage
   b. Greens
   c. Iceberg lettuce
   d. Red potatoes

12. A client is on rifampin and INH for the next 6 months. Which food would the nurse suggest the client eat more of while the client is on these medications?
   a. Kidney beans
   b. Steamed broccoli
   c. Aged cheeses with a yellow color
   d. Baked fish

13. A client is prescribed Lithobid. Which of these substances taken in excess may cause problems with the serum drug levels for the client?
   a. Tums antacid
   b. Potato chips
   c. Bananas
   d. Chocolate chip cookies

14. Which rationale is the most accurate for the nurse to teach an adolescent with Type I diabetes mellitus?
   a. Some days insulin needs are minimal only if your diet is decreased.
   b. The beta cells have stopped production of plasma insulin.
   c. Some parts of the pancreas have become nonfunctional and scarred.
   d. As you get older you may gain weight with the progressive decrease in the function of the pancreas.

15. Oral chelating agents run the risk of transient changes in which of these lab tests?
   a. Liver function
   b. Renal function
   c. Cardiac enzymes
   d. Pancreatic enzymes

16. Which sequence used by a client to draw up two types of insulin is the most recommended?
   a. Short acting then intermediate acting
   b. Intermediate acting then short acting
   c. Short acting then extended acting
   d. Regular acting then extended acting

17. The most important nurse responsibility during mannitol (Osmitrol) parenteral administration to prevent complications is to:
   a. Position clients in a prone position with the use of a deep intramuscular technique.
   b. Include an in-line filter for the prevention of foreign matter distribution.
   c. Monitor blood pressure every 15 minutes for 1 hour.
   d. Evaluate the effectiveness of renal function for increases in urine output.

18. Phenobarbital is ordered for a child with the dosage of "15 mg BID." The pharmacy label reads "each tablet = ¼ Gr." What action should the nurse take?
   a. Dispense one tablet twice a day.
   b. Dispense two tablets twice a day.
   c. Return the drug to the pharmacy with a request for the appropriate tablet dosage.

d. Return the drug to the pharmacy with a request for a liquid form of the medication.

19. A client, who had visited the health center with concerns about having venereal disease, is diagnosed with syphilis. The order is written to give 2.4 million units of benzathine penicillin. What nursing action associated with medication administration is indicated at the onset of the client-nurse interaction?

a. Tell the client about a delay since you questioned the order for excessive dosage.

b. Discuss the client's previous experience with injections.

c. Inform the client of a need to give the dose in two injections, one in each buttock, as the client lies in a prone position with supination of the feet.

d. Ask about an allergy history related to sulfa drugs.

20. In situations with an ingestion of hydrocarbons by a child the nurse plans to question which of these substances if ordered?

a. Syrup of ipecac

b. Milk

c. Oxygen via mask

d. Intravenous cephalosporin

21. Which of these findings indicate complications from a 6-day post-acetaminophen (Tylenol) overdose?

a. Liver tenderness

b. A decreasing serum ALT

c. A slightly sustained level of an elevated prothrombin time

d. Further elevation of the serum AST

22. What is the major physiological problem arising from the overuse of Epsom salts by a client?

a. Minimal spontaneous intestinal peristalsis

b. Thinning of the intestinal mucosa

c. Imbalance of acid in the stomach

d. Altered absorption of protein-like nutrients

23. A client has a history of heroin addiction. For which of these problems would this client be least likely screened?

a. Anemia

b. Syphilis

c. Tuberculosis

d. Symptomatic bacteremia

24. In clients with which of these diagnoses would the nurse decide that instruction about aspirin is a priority?

a. Osteoarthritis

b. Coronary artery disease

c. Rheumatoid arthritis

d. Lupus erythematosus

25. A client reports to have blood pressure controlled by medication. However, the client questions why there is a need to continue the medication when no feelings of sickness are experienced. The best response by the nurse is which of these comments?

a. "Your medicine keeps your blood pressure at a lower level."

b. "Your brain, heart, and kidneys are prevented from being damaged as you take the medicine to keep your blood pressure within normal ranges."

c. "If your pressure is sustained within normal ranges, eventually you may be weaned off the medication.

d. "With weight loss, regular exercise, and a very low-sodium diet, you may be able to come off the medication."

26. Oxytocin (Pitocin) administration to augment labor may result in fetal trauma from which of these effects?
    a. Precipitous delivery
    b. Uterine stimulation
    c. Tetany of the uterus
    d. Water intoxication

27. A client with a prescription of hydrocortisone sodium succinate (Solu-Cortef) requires the same instruction as a client who is taking which of these medications?
    a. Vasopressin
    b. Methimazole (Tapazole)
    c. Somatrem (Protropin)
    d. Dexamethasone (Decadron)

28. Which of these drugs is used to prevent further pathology that contributes to cerebral vascular accidents?
    a. Ticlopidine (Ticlid)
    b. Streptokinase (Streptase)
    c. Heparin sodium
    d. Aminocaproic acid (Amicar)

29. One of the adverse effects of antilipemic agents requires which lab values to be monitored every few months for changes?
    a. PT, aPTT
    b. ALT, AST
    c. LDH, alkaline phosphate
    d. Ammonia level, AST

30. Which of these drugs directly relaxes skeletal muscles by decreasing the availability of calcium in the muscle?
    a. Diazepam (Valium)
    b. Carisoprodol (Soma)
    c. Cyclobenzaprine HCl (Flexeril)
    d. Dantrolene sodium (Dantrium)

31. Vitamin B_6 is advised to protect the nervous system when the client is taking which of these drugs?
    a. Benztropine (Cogentin)
    b. Rifampin
    c. Levodopa
    d. Neostigmine methylsulfate (Prostigmin)

32. Which of these agents usually requires the addition of anticholinergic drugs to control any extrapyramidal effects?
    a. Antianxiety
    b. Antiparkinsonian
    c. Antipsychotic
    d. Psychotropics

33. Hypotension as a consequence of spinal anesthesia has a physiology of which of these origins?
    a. Catecholamine release
    b. Histamine response
    c. Sympathetic blockade
    d. Parasympathetic blockade

34. Which intervention, upon completion of the admission assessment, is most indicated for a client who had an acute head injury?
    a. Maintain the client in a resting position
    b. Provide for mouth care every hour and PRN
    c. Implement activities to prevent increases in intracranial pressure
    d. Prevent constipation

35. In preparing a client for a femoral arteriogram, the nurse should provide the client with which of these facts?
    a. The dye will be removed prior to the return to your room.
    b. The dye will cause feelings of nausea at the time of injection and for the remainder of the day.
    c. A regional anesthetic will be given to decrease your sensation of pain at the insertion site of the catheter.
    d. A local anesthetic is injected into the insertion site to diminish any discomfort.
36. A client is scheduled for a 12-lead electrocardiograph stress test. The client is to be advised that which of these items is needed during the test?
    a. A pair of sturdy slippers
    b. Walking shoes
    c. A clean pair of socks
    d. Hospital coverlets for shoes as used in the surgical suite
37. A client diagnosed with cancer is on therapy of filgrastim (Neupogen), a colony-stimulating factor. Which of these medications is the best to administer?
    a. Aspirin
    b. Acetaminophen
    c. Meperidine HCl
    d. MS Contin
38. A client with heart failure is monitored for the effectiveness of a dose of furosemide (Lasix). Changes in which of these parameters is most

likely the earliest to be reported to the physician as a reflection that the total volume pumped through the heart is different?
    a. Central venous pressure
    b. Peripheral arterial pressure
    c. Pulse oximeter reading
    d. Heart rate
39. If the client on peripheral hyperalimentation has the IV infiltrated and discontinued, which of these manifestations is to be anticipated within the initial 2 hours of infiltration?
    a. Lethargy, sleepiness
    b. Agitation, coordination of motor skills
    c. Confusion, insomnia
    d. Restlessness, irritability
40. The nurse is calling a client at home to schedule a morning electroencephalogram in 48 hours. What advice should the nurse give the client?
    a. Take nothing by mouth for 12 to 14 hours before the exam.
    b. Omit coffee for a minimum of 24 hours prior to the exam.
    c. Withhold your anticonvulsant until after the test is completed.
    d. Take your anticonvulsant with a sip of water on the morning of the test and do not eat or drink anything else.
41. A client with acquired immunodeficiency syndrome complains of persistent diarrhea, muscle cramps, constant dizziness after initially standing, and sluggishness. These data support which priority nursing diagnosis for this client?
    a. Risk for infection
    b. Altered nutrition, less than body requirements

c. Fluid volume deficit

d. Impaired perianal skin integrity

42. A preschooler with multi–drug-resistant tuberculosis makes the following statements. Which statement indicates a need for further teaching?

a. "When I stop coughing up stuff, I can go outside of my room."

b. "I probably have to take this medicine for a long time, maybe until I go into the kindergarten."

c. "When I must cough, I can use my tissue or a handkerchief."

d. "I can eat oatmeal with walnuts every day."

43. A client with esophagitis is prescribed the dopamine antagonist metoclopramide HCl (Reglan). The nurse should explain that this medication is given for which of these reasons?

a. Increases the resting tone of the lower esophageal sphincter

b. Acts as a gastric stimulant and mucosal antiinflammatory

c. Increases gastric motility with stimulation of gastric secretions

d. Protects the gastric mucosa

44. A client is stabilized on a lithium dose. Which of these actions by the client is most dangerous to the client?

a. The client misses the lab checks for lithium levels every other month.

b. The client reports not cooking with or adding salt to food.

c. The client makes a remark about the need to drink a can of regular soda every hour while at work.

d. The client plans to have a child some time in the future.

45. During a home visit a client is taught how to irrigate a colostomy. While practicing the irrigation procedure the client has difficulty in catheter insertion. Which action should the nurse take?

a. Help the client with the procedure.

b. Guide the client to use a little Vaseline on the tip of the catheter prior to insertion.

c. Direct the client to gently dilate the stoma with a water-soluble lubricated, gloved finger.

d. Suggest the client insert a glycerine suppository 10 minutes prior to irrigation to moisten the intestinal mucosa

46. A middle-aged female client receives daily these medications: enalapril (Vasotec), estrogen, progestin, lithium carbonate, and lorazepam. Which of these groups of findings should alert the nurse for medication interactions?

a. Recent memory loss, muscle weakness, hyperreflexia

b. Blood pressure 142/90, reports of mood swings, restless night sleep

c. Slight kyphosis, occasional hot flashes, heavier menstrual flow

d. Feelings of panic and anxiety, occasional loss of train of thought during conversations, sleepiness

47. A client is scheduled for an electromyography 3 days from now. The nurse calls the client to confirm the appointment and to give information about client needs during this procedure. The nurse should include which of these items during the conversation?
    a. Avoid drinking or eating for 8 hours prior to the test.
    b. Omit any scheduled diazepam (Valium) for 24 hours prior to the procedure.
    c. Expect to feel very little to no pain during the procedure.
    d. Practice lying still since the client will need to remain still during the procedure.

48. A nurse prepares to draw up 50 mg of a 100 mg ampule of a narcotic analgesic. The nurse should know that the unused portion of the medication should be:
    a. Placed in the refrigerator with the label clearly marked with the client's name and room number, date, and time opened.
    b. Returned to the pharmacy and credited to the client's account.
    c. Returned to the locked cabinet to be used the next time the client is in pain.
    d. Disposed of into the sink while in the presence of another licensed staff member and documented in the record.

49. A client questions why anti-gout medication has been included in the chemotherapy regimen. The nurse should include teaching that these medications given in conjunction with chemotherapy have what action?
    a. Enhance the effects of the antineoplastic agents
    b. Decrease the side effect of nausea
    c. Prevent findings of gout that may occur from rapid cell destruction
    d. Protect normal cells from destruction by the promotion of folic acid conversion

50. Anticholinergics are given prior to surgical procedures to dry oral and respiratory secretions. These effects reduce the risk of aspiration and airway irritability. Anticholinergics are also given for which of these purposes of prevention?
    a. Nausea
    b. Cardiac arrhythmia
    c. Urinary retention
    d. Respiratory depression

51. Histamine H_2 receptor blocking agents have which of these primary effects?
    a. Neutralize stomach acid
    b. Protect stomach mucosa
    c. Prevent gastric acid secretion
    d. Increase gastric peristalsis

52. Erythromycin ointment rather than silver nitrate ointment is used in the prophylactic eye care of a newborn. The nurse explains to the mother that which of these effects supports this choice of treatment?
    a. It promotes a longer bacteriostatic effect
    b. A more rapid systemic effect is obtained
    c. Therapeutic amounts are administered easier
    d. Minimal irritation of the conjunctiva occurs

53. A 6-year-old child with cardiac defects has had a cardiac catheterization for a third time. For the first few hours after the procedure, which of these actions should the nurse implement as the priority?
    a. Keep the head of the bed elevated 30 degrees
    b. Check the child's blood pressure every hour
    c. Monitor the child's bilateral distal pulses in the extremities
    d. Have the child cough forcefully at regular intervals

54. Discharge instructions are given to the parents of a 3-year-old who is started on digoxin twice a day. The least desirable data to give during teaching are which of these items?
    a. Do not mix or give the medication with food.
    b. Hold the medicine if the child's heart rate is below 100 beats per minute.
    c. Call the physician's office if the child has nausea and vomiting.
    d. If the dose is missed, give it as soon as possible then readjust the 12-hour interval of administration.

55. A client is receiving thrombolytic and anticoagulant therapy for an acute myocardial infarction. Which of these findings should be reported to the physician before the physician's regularly scheduled rounds?
    a. Hematuria
    b. Isolated premature ventricular contractions

c. A change in heart rate from 120 to 80
d. An increase in the client's pain relief

56. The nurse should instruct clients who take thiazide drugs to include foods in their diet that are high in which of these substances?
    a. Calcium
    b. Iron
    c. Protein
    d. Magnesium

57. A 2-year-old child in the acute phase of nephrotic syndrome has the following findings. Which should the nurse be most concerned about and report to the physician?
    a. Ate less of each meal over the past 24 hours
    b. Is easily fatigued and lethargic
    c. Has a cloudy nasal discharge
    d. Has edema of the genital area

58. A client is prescribed both a broad-spectrum antibiotic and a sulfonamide. Which of these actions is most essential in this client's daily care?
    a. Weighing and observing for edema or rashes
    b. Giving extra fluids and monitoring urine output
    c. Taking the client's blood pressure at regular intervals
    d. Evaluating the client frequently for findings of photophobia and hyperreflexia

59. An elderly client has been taking Azulfidine for more than a week. Which of these findings if reported

by this client is a priority concern and needs to be reported to the physician?

a. Severe back pain on one side
b. Epigastric pain of increased frequency
c. Severe, cramping pain in the left upper quadrant especially 2 to 3 hours after eating
d. Some dizziness when first standing but it subsides quickly and often doesn't occur if the client gets up slowly

60. A newborn is to receive medication via a gastric tube. In determination of the catheter placement, which of these actions is the most desirable for the nurse to use?

a. Insert the tip of a large syringe into the catheter and withdraw an amount of air equal to the amount of the feeding.
b. Insert a few drops of sterile water or saline into the catheter, hold the end of the catheter below the level of the stomach, and observe for drainage of gastric contents.
c. Inject about 0.5 to 1.0 ml of air into the catheter during which time the nurse listens over the infant's abdomen with a stethoscope for the entry point of the air bolus.
d. Insert about 5.0 ml of sterile water or saline into the catheter and observe the infant's respirations.

61. A 35-year-old female is hospitalized for a cerebral bleed into the circle of Willis. The physician has prescribed oxygen per nasal cannula and man- nitol intravenously. The nurse should give the mannitol with the knowledge that it:

a. Delays seizure activity.
b. Decreases any swelling in the brain.
c. Constricts the affected cerebral arteries.
d. Decreases inflammation.

62. An elderly client visits the local health clinic for findings of vesicles and a rash on the right cheek. The client is diagnosed with herpes zoster with involvement of the trigeminal nerve on the right side of the face. Prescriptions include acetaminophen (Tylenol). During further assessment of the client it would be important for the nurse to obtain the answer to which of these questions?

a. Has the client been exposed to anyone with chickenpox?
b. Does the client have a history of developing canker sores?
c. Is the client using a new shaving cream?
d. Has the client ever had a dermatologic reaction to food?

63. A client is scheduled for an ultra- sonography for cholelithiasis. Prior to this procedure the clinic nurse anticipates:

a. Administering a sedative about 30 to 45 minutes before the actual procedure.
b. Questioning the client about allergies to iodine and seafood.
c. Keeping the client NPO.
d. Explaining the procedure and its purpose.

64. A client diagnosed with chronic renal failure asks why the physician prescribed aluminum hydroxide gel. The nurse should explain that the expected action of the drug is which of these actions?
    a. To aid in inhibition of the secretion of hydrochloric acid
    b. To serve as a catalyst in the breakdown of proteins
    c. To neutralize gastric secretions
    d. To aid in the excretion of phosphate

65. A narcotic and a nonnarcotic analgesic are both ordered every 3 to 4 hours for a postoperative client of 16 hours. When the nurse makes rounds the client complains of the severe pain returning. The nurse checks the medication record to see that the client had the narcotic 3 hours ago. Which of these actions would be most appropriate for the nurse to take initially?
    a. Reposition the client.
    b. Give the client a back rub.
    c. Administer the prescribed narcotic analgesic.
    d. Administer the prescribed nonnarcotic analgesic.

66. Because a client was in a lithotomy position for a prolonged period of time during a procedure, the nurse should perform which of these actions during the early postprocedure period?
    a. Turn the client from side to side with a pillow placed between the client's legs.
    b. Encourage flexion and extension exercises of the legs and apply elastic stockings.
    c. Elevate the foot of the bed to 15 degrees and put a pillow at the head of the bed.
    d. Place the bed in reverse Trendelenburg position and put a pillow at the foot of the bed.

67. In developing care plans for clients in the age group of 90 to 100 years, the nurse should include gradual supervised ambulation, especially after procedures, to:
    a. Shift the center of gravity in the body forward.
    b. Promote use of extensor rather than flexor muscles.
    c. Minimize the response to orthostatic reflex stimulation.
    d. Deter ossification of the long bones.

68. A client is prescribed methantheline bromide (Banthine) for the treatment of ulcerative colitis. The nurse should explain to the client that the chief purpose of this drug is to:
    a. Suppress inflammation of the bowel wall.
    b. Reduce peristaltic activity.
    c. Neutralize gastrointestinal tract acidity.
    d. Minimize feelings of anxiety.

69. The nurse has to do a heel stick on a newborn. Which aspect of the heel should the nurse select?
    a. Lateral
    b. Medial
    c. Distal
    d. Dorsal

70. A client has an infusion of D_5 0.45 normal saline at 125 ml/hour through an infusion pump. Which of these actions by a student nurse is of a concern to the charge nurse?
    a. Checks that the volume infused coincides with the tape on the intravenous bottle
    b. Adjusts the height of the pump attachment to ensure that the intravenous fluid flows by gravity
    c. Checks that the intravenous tubes are not pinched or kinked
    d. Includes the type of infusion device in the documentation on the medication record

71. An adult client is placed on amoxicillin therapy. To detect untoward effects of this medication the nurse should teach the client to report which of these findings as initial subtle manifestations of problems with this medication?
    a. Frequent loose stools
    b. Difficulty with breathing
    c. Generalized dermatitis
    d. An itching rash on the abdomen

72. An adolescent was admitted with vomiting, diarrhea, and gastrointestinal bleeding. The physician orders an infusion of lactated Ringer's with potassium chloride. The nurse should explain to the client that the infusion is given for which purpose?
    a. Replenishment of the electrolytes lost through the bleeding
    b. Restoration of the fluids and potassium lost with the gastrointestinal losses

    c. Provision of potassium to promote the retention of fluid to combat the dehydration
    d. Furnish potassium for the minimization of intestinal cramping and colic

73. A nurse is to select a site for the administration of parenteral drugs for a client with second- and third-degree burns. It is essential that the nurse consider which of these consequences associated with the client's injury?
    a. Impaired circulation hampers drug absorption.
    b. Decreased blood volume shortens the period of drug action.
    c. Drug action is potentiated by increased blood viscosity.
    d. Concentration of blood plasma in the tissues potentiates the desired effects of the drug.

74. Tamoxifen citrate 10 mg PO BID was prescribed for your client. Which of these findings indicates an adverse effect?
    a. Bone pain
    b. Insomnia
    c. Anorexia
    d. Purpura on the legs

75. An adolescent is taking 0.125 mg of digoxin daily. Which condition could most likely predispose the client to develop digitalis toxicity?
    a. Hypomagnesemia
    b. Hyperkalemia
    c. Hypothyroidism
    d. Hyperparathyroidism

76. Neupogen 200 mg units subcutaneously is given daily for 7 days to a client. Which of these laboratory reports should the nurse monitor after these injections?
   a. Red blood cell counts
   b. White blood cell counts
   c. Platelets
   d. Sedimentation rates

77. A client has received streptomycin for over 6 weeks. The nurse should monitor this client for which side effect?
   a. Hepatitis
   b. Arthralgia
   c. Ototoxicity
   d. Neurotoxicity

78. After 1 year of taking antitubercular drug therapy the client should be advised by the nurse to have the serum enzymes checked for which of these systems?
   a. Pancreatic
   b. Liver
   c. Gastric
   d. Cardiac

79. Disulfiram is prescribed for a client recovering from alcoholism. The nurse should teach the client to avoid which of these substances?
   a. Elixir of terpin hydrate
   b. Aspirin
   c. Benadryl
   d. Tylenol

80. Which of these environmental factors would the nurse expect to be the most disturbing to a client who develops delirium tremens?
   a. A bright room
   b. A dark room
   c. Medicinal odors
   d. Odors from fragrances

81. The nurse administers a pancreatin replacement to a child. The nurse should expect that the most important outcome of this treatment is increased absorption of which of these substances?
   a. Proteins
   b. Fats
   c. Carbohydrates
   d. Folic and ascorbic acids

82. A client has had a transection of the spinal cord at the T4 level. Rehabilitation includes the use of leg braces. When applying and removing the leg braces it is a priority for the nurse to consider if the client has which of these manifestations?
   a. Cannot move either lower extremity
   b. Has minimal flexion of the knees
   c. Cannot fully extend the hip joints
   d. Has no sensation in the lower extremities

83. A client is prescribed a regimen of these drugs: cyclophosphamide, methotrexate, and fluorouracil. Which item needs to be included in this client's education plan while the client is taking these medications?
   a. An increase in fluids to 3 to 4 liters per day is required.
   b. Protection from direct sun exposure is crucial.
   c. Foods that are sweet are better tolerated for nausea control and prevention.
   d. A regimen of lying down every 2 hours is recommended to prevent postural hypotension.

84. A client with terminal lung cancer is being treated at home with a morphine drip for intractable pain. Which of these findings should the nurse recognize as a complication of this medication regimen?
    a. The client requires minimal rescue doses of pain medication.
    b. The family reports that the client has had frequent, small, liquid stools over the past week.
    c. The client's respirations are deep, restful, and at a rate of 10.
    d. The client's heart rate is recorded to range from 50 to 94.

85. A client is admitted from an extended care facility with the diagnosis of multiple drug-resistant tuberculosis. The nurse expects to find which of these notations in the documentation received from the facility?
    a. Crackles, cyanosis, fever
    b. Persistent fever, weight loss, night sweats
    c. Sudden chest pain, hemoptysis, heart rate of 138
    d. Nausea, diaphoresis, severe chest pain

86. A client with moderate preeclampsia is placed on an external fetal monitor. Moderate uterine contractions are occurring every 4 minutes and are 45 to 50 seconds in duration. In view of this situation, which of these findings should the nurse consider ominous and report to the midwife immediately?
    a. Urine output hourly sequence of 60 ml, 25 ml, 30 ml, and 25 ml
    b. A change of protein from 1+ to 2+ in the client's urine

    c. Generalized edema with no further increase
    d. Complaints of right-upper quadrant discomfort with severe epigastric pain

87. A client is discussing the preparation for an upper gastrointestinal series of x-rays. Which of these statements by the client indicates both accurate and appropriate expectations?
    a. "In the testing department I will be asked to drink a liquid similar to a milk shake. Then a series of pictures will be taken over a few hours."
    b. "I will be asked to swallow a tube after I drink a thick liquid. X-rays will be taken during the time I swallow the liquid and the tube."
    c. "I expect to drink a substance that is radioactive. Pictures of my stomach will be taken in a series. I will be able to be around my family 3 hours after the test when the radioactivity is gone."
    d. "I will have pictures taken of my swallowing a thick milk shake liquid."

88. A few hours after delivery a newborn is observed to be lethargic with a generalized dusky skin tone. This infant is from a mother with gestational diabetes mellitus. The nurse should recognize that the newborn has manifestations of which imbalance?
    a. Hypercalcemia
    b. Hypokalemia
    c. Hypoglycemia
    d. Hypoxemia

89. Ninety minutes ago a client's oxygen concentration via mask was changed to 40% from 50%. The arterial blood gas results have changed in that the arterial oxygen pressure value has decreased by 20% to 50 mm Hg. Which action should the nurse take?
    a. Continue to monitor the client since the drop in arterial oxygen pressure is an expected outcome from the decrease in oxygen concentration via mask.
    b. Increase the oxygen concentration to what it was prior to the decrease to 40%.
    c. Increase the oxygen concentration and repeat the blood gases in an hour.
    d. Further evaluate the client for changes and inform the physician of all findings.

90. A client is admitted to an alcoholic treatment center. The client has been drinking in excess of a quart of liquor a day for 5 to 7 years. The client has been drinking up until the time of admission. The orders include a regimen for a diet as tolerated, thiamine injection daily × 3, and a tranquilizer q 4 hours by mouth. The nurse should anticipate that this client is susceptible to delirium tremens during which of these time frames?
    a. Within the initial hours of hospitalization
    b. Between 48 and 72 hours of the initial hospitalization

    c. Minimal risk of delirium tremens since the client will receive thiamine
    d. A relatively minimal risk of delirium tremens for this client between 24 and 72 hours of the initial hospitalization

91. A client with prolonged intravenous therapy has an implanted venous access device. The nurse prepares to insert a specially designed needle to institute a continuous infusion of fluids. At what angle should the nurse insert this needle into the venous access device?
    a. 15 degrees
    b. 30 degrees
    c. 45 degrees
    d. 90 degrees

92. A client is started on central total parenteral nutrition. Which of these nursing procedures has the highest priority?
    a. Blood pressure and heart rate every 2 to 4 hours
    b. Peripheral blood glucose monitoring every hour
    c. Daily weights
    d. Level of consciousness every 2 to 3 hours

93. A client is diagnosed with acute bronchial pneumonia. Which of these medications would the nurse anticipate teaching the client about during the hospital stay?
    a. Erythromycin
    b. Adrenalin
    c. Rifampin
    d. Aminophylline

94. The nurse would advise the mother of which of these children to have a booster dose of tetanus toxoid since all children have completed their primary tetanus immunization within the past 5 years?
    a. The child who is having dental treatment for an abscessed impacted molar
    b. The child who stubs the big toe and has a large hematoma, or "blood blister," under the skin
    c. The child who gets a cut from a broken bottle while walking barefoot on the beach
    d. The child who sustains several long scratches on bare legs while climbing over a wooden fence in the backyard
95. Which of these dietary modifications should the nurse recommend to a client who reports findings of dumping syndrome?
    a. Minimize the fat intake
    b. Restrict the animal protein intake
    c. Increase the total number of calories
    d. Decrease the intake of concentrated carbohydrates
96. After bladder reconstruction surgery the physician prescribes belladonna and opium suppositories to minimize the client's bladder spasms. Which of these notations on the chart should alert the nurse to hold the initial dose and notify the physician?
    a. History of peptic ulcers
    b. Occasional migraine headaches

c. Client may self-administer miotic eye drops for glaucoma
    d. Petit mal seizures during the teen years
97. A client is receiving 500 mg of aminophylline in 1000 ml of normal saline at 25 ml per hour. The morning serum aminophylline level is 24. What should the nurse do?
    a. Nothing since this is within therapeutic range
    b. Notify the physician
    c. Decrease the rate of infusion by 10%
    d. Notify the physician to request a repeat blood level in 2 hours
98. The nurse is giving massive amounts of fluids to a client in shock. When the nurse notes which of these changes should the nurse increase the fluids and notify the physician that the client is progressing further into the shock state?
    a. A increase in the heart rate from 120 to 130
    b. A sustained decrease in urine output from 30 ml to 25 ml per hour
    c. A change in the blood pressure from 100/60 to 88/58
    d. A rise in respiratory rate to 36 from 28
99. The physician orders a purified protein derivative test on a client who the nurse suspects is anergic. The nurse anticipates that the reaction to this test is most likely to be which of these findings?
    a. Negative reaction
    b. A >10 mm induration
    c. A <10 mm induration
    d. A >15 mm induration

100. A nurse in the endoscopic lab is preparing a client with chronic liver failure and ascites for an abdominal paracentesis. The nurse must include which of these actions?
    a. Instruct the client on how to participate in the procedure
    b. Have the client in a dangling position on the side of the bed
    c. Have the client empty the bladder just prior to the procedure
    d. Provide the client with a rolled blanket to place against the back while the client maintains a sitting or side-lying position during the procedure

101. The most common cause of leg cramps for a client who takes loop diuretics is which of these low values?
    a. Potassium
    b. Magnesium
    c. Calcium
    d. Protein

102. A client has started on broad-spectrum antibiotics. The nurse instructs the client that the medicine is effective if which of these occurs?
    a. The passage of normal stool instead of diarrhea
    b. The prior pain is relieved
    c. The temperature drops 2 degrees
    d. The urine is clear with a pungent odor

103. The nurse should remember that clients with asthma:
    a. Should restrict fluid intake.
    b. Have attacks that are brought on by anxiety.
    c. May have difficulty coughing up sputum.
    d. Will improve quickly with hospitalization.

104. A client states, "I can't catch my breath." The best position for this client is:
    a. Prone.
    b. Supine.
    c. Trendelenburg.
    d. Whatever position the client prefers.

105. To evaluate the progress of a client with asthma, which variable would provide the best information about the client's overall condition?
    a. Respiratory rate
    b. Breath sounds
    c. Respiratory effort
    d. Inspiratory/expiratory ratio

106. A postoperative client complains about pain in the abdomen. To compare the current level of pain with previous reports of pain the nurse should:
    a. Use a pain scale.
    b. Use a subjective scale.
    c. Ask the client, "Is it more or less?"
    d. See how much pain medication the client has received.

107. A client with a diagnosis of glomerular nephritis treated by a sulfonamide has an order to force liquids. When the lunch tray comes the client asks for something more to drink. The nurse should encourage the client to drink:
    a. Water.
    b. Apple juice.
    c. Orange juice.
    d. Hot chocolate.

108. When performing a routine dressing change around a new tracheostomy, using standard precautions, the nurse would use:
    a. Gloves and goggles.
    b. A gown and gloves.
    c. A mask with an eye shield and gloves.
    d. A gown and face mask.
109. The nurse would advance a client on a clear liquid diet when the client:
    a. Is hungry.
    b. Is fully ambulatory.
    c. Has the IV removed.
    d. Can tolerate clear liquids.
110. A child is admitted with the diagnosis of leukemia. In a review of this client's lab results, the nurse would expect to see:
    a. A low potassium level.
    b. Bacteria in the urine.
    c. A high glucose level.
    d. A low platelet count.
111. A client is 6 years old. During the provision of care the nurse should consider this client's development to recognize that:
    a. The child needs to be like his/her peers.
    b. Separation anxiety is at its peak.
    c. The child has an increased need for privacy.
    d. The child's fears about his/her body changing are greater than his/her fear of being apart from his/her parents.
112. The physician has ordered a test to help confirm the diagnosis of leukemia. The nurse would expect to prepare the client for:
    a. An MRI.
    b. A chest x-ray.
    c. A lumbar puncture.
    d. A bone marrow aspiration.
113. One of the goals of a child's care is that he remains free of infection. To evaluate if this goal has been met, the nurse would observe for:
    a. Increased urine output.
    b. Normal body temperature.
    c. Fewer visits from the child's parents.
    d. A change in the child's white blood cell count.
114. When the nurse listens to the fetal heartbeat during a mother's 7-month visit, what rate would be expected?
    a. 90 beats/ minute
    b. 110 beats/ minute
    c. 140 beats/ minute
    d. 170 beats/ minute
115. In helping a mother set long-term goals for her baby's care, the nurse should plan to emphasize the need for the mother to:
    a. Plan time to sleep.
    b. Find a place to live.
    c. Learn about proper baby care.
    d. Identify community resources.
116. In helping a pregnant client choose proper foods during pregnancy, the nurse should advise her that she:
    a. Will need extra calcium daily.
    b. May have a beer once every 2 weeks.
    c. Should decrease her fluid intake in the evening.
    d. Might have food cravings that indicate nutritional deficiencies.

117. A pregnant mother has attended childbirth classes. The statement by her that shows an understanding of childbirth instructions would be:
    a. "I'll be knocked out with narcotics."
    b. "I'll be all by myself and doing all the work during labor."
    c. "Breathing can help with the pain."
    d. "I can have all the pain medicine in my epidural that I want."

118. A client was admitted to the mental health unit because voices are telling him to stab his neighbor. The statement by this client that indicates a potential for danger and needs to be reported to the charge nurse is:
    a. "I want to see my daughter."
    b. "The voices are telling me to stop eating."
    c. "I want to take a shower and shave."
    d. "I will do whatever the voices say."

119. A client is diagnosed with schizophrenia. As his condition improves the nurse should:
    a. Offer a rigid schedule to provide him with structure.
    b. Offer two or three choices so as not to overwhelm him.
    c. Offer no choices because he is incapable of decision-making.
    d. Offer him a range of choices so that he can select activities he is really interested in.

120. When a client has auditory hallucinations, the nurse's best action is to tell the client:
    a. They simply don't exist.
    b. He must prove the voices are real.
    c. To get involved in a unit-based activity.
    d. You can imagine the voices are frightening.

121. Side effects of the antipsychotic medication Thorazine (chlorpromazine HCl) that the nurse should observe for include:
    a. Nausea.
    b. Drowsiness.
    c. Hypertension.
    d. Frequent urination.

122. The nurse would expect a client with pulmonary edema to cough up sputum that is:
    a. Red or pink and frothy.
    b. Clear or white and thin.
    c. Brown or gray and plug-like.
    d. Yellow or green and thick.

123. A client is to be discharged on scheduled doses of morphine sulfate by the intravenous route. The client has been on this medication for 2 weeks while in the hospital. Which of these foods is good to recommend, so as not to cause medication side effects?
    a. Bran cereal with milk
    b. Rice cereal with milk
    c. Peanut butter sandwiches
    d. Cheese sandwiches

124. A client in the radiology room for an MRI becomes very anxious and refuses the procedure. Which of

these actions is most appropriate for the nurse to do at this time?
a. Advise the client that the family can stay in the room during the MRI.
b. Tell the client to wait 5 minutes to get less anxious since the procedure is not painful.
c. Notify the physician of the client's refusal.
d. Have the client reschedule the procedure.

125. Of four mental health clients, the client with which diagnosis would have the priority to be admitted to a private room?
a. Obsessive-compulsive
b. Depression
c. Bipolar
d. Borderline personality

126. A client who has a recent left below the knee amputation is reported to be independent per activities and receiving O₂ at 3 liters per minute. Which of these actions is a priority for the client's ambulation during the night?
a. Have the call light within reach of the client.
b. Ensure the bed is in a low position.
c. Turn the night light on in the room.
d. Extend the oxygen tubing.

127. During the admission of a toddler to the pediatric unit the priority of the admissions nurse is obtain a history of the child's:
a. Daytime routine.
b. Toilet training.
c. Communication style.
d. Bedtime routine.

128. The most important aspect of hand-washing is which of these items?
a. Soap
b. Friction
c. Paper towels
d. Warm water

129. Dobutamine 250 mg in 500 ml is mixed and ready for infusion for maintenance therapy. The client weighs 60 kg. The physician has ordered 3 μg/kg/min. What sequence of actions should the nurse do?
a. Check the client's blood pressure and the heart rate, start the infusion, recheck the blood and heart rate in 15 minutes.
b. Check the client's respiratory rate and effort, start the infusion, recheck these parameters in 15 minutes.
c. Check the client's vital signs, start the infusion only if the blood pressure <90 systolic.
d. Check the earlier blood pressure and heart rate, start the infusion, recheck the blood and heart rate in 1 hour.

130. A child is admitted with the diagnosis of leukemia. In a review of this client's lab results, the nurse would expect to see:
a. A high potassium level.
b. A high white count.
c. A low glucose level.
d. A high platelet count.

131. The physician has ordered an invasive test to help confirm the diagnosis of leukemia. After the procedure the nurse would expect to care

for a dressing located where on the client?

a. The flank
b. The right upper quadrant of the abdomen
c. The lower lumbar area
d. The iliac crest

132. A client is scheduled for a liver biopsy in 2 days. The pretest lab work has been returned to the outpatient office. Which of these reports would the nurse be sure to notify the physician of by the end of the day?

a. Hemoglobin of 10.5
b. Activated partial thromboplastin time of 45
c. Elevated blood urea nitrogen
d. Elevated ammonia level

133. The nurse has received the evening report about 10 clients. Of the clients with these situations, which client would the nurse assign to the patient care technician?

a. Post-cardiac catheterization
b. Post-computerized tomogram
c. Pregnant client with hypertension
d. Pre-biopsy of the breast

134. Which of these side effects is the nurse to monitor for in a 4-year-old who takes tricyclics?

a. Bradycardia
b. Wetting of the bed
c. Hyperactivity
d. Hypertension

135. Which of these actions is essential for the nurse to teach a client who is prescribed Synthroid?

a. Monitor for persistent constipation
b. Note changes in sleep patterns

c. Daily pulse checks prior to getting out of bed in the morning
d. Observe for changes in energy levels

136. Which of these factors might make an elderly client prone to accidents?

a. Decreased ability to recall
b. Inability to reason
c. Altered nutritional status
d. Decreased sensory acuity

137. Which of these foods is to be encouraged to be taken minimally by clients with renal failure?

a. Apples
b. Dried fruit
c. Cranberries
d. Apricots

138. The registered nurse has received the evening report for the team. Which of these clients would the nurse go to first?

a. A client screaming of pain
b. A client with a beeping IV pump
c. A client who put the light on to tell that the drainage on the dressing had increased
d. A client the family reported had a reaction to the medication yesterday

139. Which of these foods has the most protein?

a. Chicken broth
b. A medium potato
c. A medium avocado
d. Tapioca pudding

140. If you saw a nurse perform these actions, which one requires you to notify the charge nurse?

a. Auscultate lung sounds in a sequence of right to left
b. Give atropine for sinus tachycardia

c. Give an IM injection with a 1-inch 25 gauge needle

d. Withdraw Humulin-N insulin after rotating and not rolling the bottle

141. Which roommate would you choose for a child with leukemia?
    a. A teenager with leukemia
    b. A child with suspected tuberculosis
    c. A toddler with intestinal inflammation
    d. A child with influenza

142. The registered nurse has received the evening report for the team. Which of these clients would the nurse assign the patient care technician to go take the vital signs of first?
    a. A client screaming of pain
    b. A client with a beeping IV pump
    c. A client who put the light on to tell that the drainage on the dressing had increased
    d. A client the family reported had a reaction to the medication on the last shift

143. Which of these clients is it most appropriate for the charge nurse to assign the patient care assistant to?
    a. A client who needs a dressing change
    b. A client with a 2-hour turning schedule
    c. A client who has returned from an x-ray procedure
    d. A client to be discharged that day

144. Which of these positions for a liver biopsy is appropriate for a client with severe COPD?
    a. A right side lying position
    b. A left side lying position
    c. A dorsal recumbent position with the right arm behind the head—low Fowler's position
    d. A dorsal recumbent position with the right arm behind the head—very low Fowler's position

145. Which of these lab results need to be monitored after injection therapy for lead poisoning in a child?
    a. Liver studies
    b. Cardiac enzymes
    c. Renal filtration rate studies
    d. Coagulation profiles

146. Therapy for the client diagnosed with a bipolar disorder is aimed at end behaviors for primarily:
    a. A mild depression.
    b. A mild mania.
    c. Hypomania.
    d. Chronic controlled mania and depression.

147. A client with suspected AIDS has a Mantoux skin test read at 48 hours with these results: erythema of 10 mm with an induration of 6 mm. These results are indicative of a test that is:
    a. Negative and read too early.
    b. Negative and requires a repeat check within 72 hours.
    c. Positive but inconclusive.
    d. Positive but inconclusive because of the suspected AIDS.

148. After the nurse gets the morning report there are four things to do within the first 60 minutes of the shift. Which of these tasks is to be done first?
    a. Check a postoperative client with an IV of normal saline in a keep open rate.
    b. Change the rate of an insulin drip as ordered within the last 30 minutes.
    c. Inspect the rate of the hyperalimentation drip and glucose level in a client.
    d. Evaluate the rate of a dopamine drip for effectiveness for a client whose blood pressure and urine output has been maintained for 72 hours.

149. With closed head trauma, what would indicate increased intracranial pressure?
    a. Increased systolic pressure
    b. Increased diastolic pressure
    c. Decreased pulse with deep breath
    d. Decreased pulse with suctioning

150. Four postoperative clients with these diagnoses arrive to the nursing unit within an 8-minute period. Which client is the nurse to assess first?
    a. A cardiac cath
    b. A femoral-popliteal bypass
    c. A radial neck dissection with a laryngectomy
    d. A radial bilateral mastectomy

151. A client had radical neck surgery over 4 weeks ago. Which of these complaints by the client would most concern the nurse?

    a. Complaints of mild difficulty swallowing
    b. Reports a need for the continued use of mild analgesics
    c. States the return of a sore throat over the past 2 days
    d. Identifies a persistent feeling of pulling or neck tightness as the head is turned from side to side

152. What would be an expected finding of mitral valve stenosis?
    a. Edema
    b. Left ventricular hypertrophy
    c. Hemoptysis
    d. Dyspnea

153. What is the best method to give an antibiotic to an infant with thrush?
    a. Mix with a teaspoon of sterile water and apply with a medicine dropper
    b. Mix with the formula of one feeding and let the baby drink from the bottle
    c. Let the infant take a few sips of sterile water then apply the antibiotic with a medicine dropper
    d. Apply the antibiotic with a Q-tip

154. A 13-year-old, admitted with second-degree burns to 30% of the body, has an immunization history of receipt of all immunizations according to the recommended schedule. At this time, tetanus prophylaxis should include which item?
    a. Tetanus toxoid
    b. Tetanus immune globulin
    c. Tetanus toxoid and tetanus immune globulin
    d. No additional protection

155. A school-age child, brought to the clinic by her grandmother, has numerous burned areas over the body and a fractured left arm. The grandmother said that the child disobeyed, left the house without permission on a bike and fell in the street. The child, refusing to talk to the nurse or the grandmother, stares at the wall. All but which of these factors supports the nurse's suspicion of child abuse?
    a. The physical presentation is inconsistent with the history of events.
    b. The child is described as disobedient.
    c. A lack of warmth is exhibited between the child and grandmother.
    d. The child's disobedience suggests that discipline is appropriate.

156. A client, age 21, in acute renal failure after hemorrhage from an accident fails to respond to appropriate therapy to correct the renal failure. Urine output is 275 ml for 24 hours; creatinine is 7.2 mg/dl; and blood urea nitrogen is 90 mg/dl. Which of these indicators would the nurse expect to see as this client progresses into a chronic renal failure?
    a. Anemia
    b. Hypokalemia
    c. Diaphoresis
    d. Hypotension

157. A client aged 32 years is married with children and has a history of being treated for over 2 years for leukemia. The client is admitted with a diagnosis of pneumonia. The client talks about knowing that death is imminent. The client uses clinical terms to describe the disease process and lacks terms of personal feelings in the conversation. One day the client states, "I'm so worried." What is the best response by the nurse?
    a. "It must be frightening to know that you are dying."
    b. "You must be very uncomfortable about this."
    c. "Have you shared these feelings with your family?
    d. "Tell me exactly what things are worrying you."

158. The nurse would expect a client with pneumonia to cough up sputum that is:
    a. Red or pink and frothy.
    b. Clear or white and thin.
    c. Brown or gray and plug-like.
    d. Yellow or green and thick.

159. A client is sent home on the medication Coumadin. The nurse is at highest risk for negligence in which of these circumstances?
    a. The client does not wear the medic alert band after discharge from the hospital.
    b. The nurse failed to document dietary restrictions education.
    c. The client did not show up for the second follow-up visit.
    d. The nurse forgot to call the physician's office with the lab reports the morning of the client's discharge.

160. Which of these clients has the higher risk of cervical cancer?
    a. A 26-year-old with multiple sex partners
    b. A 30-year-old with recurrent tuberculosis
    c. A 54-year-old with a history of celibacy
    d. An 86-year-old with a history of breast cancer
161. A mother has been caring for an infant with celiac disease. How can the nurse tell that the mother is feeding the infant correctly?
    a. By the infant's height and weight
    b. By the infant's score on the developmental chart
    c. By asking the mother what she thinks
    d. By having a 72-hour dietary recall completed
162. A client is being treated for endometriosis. The nurse is prepared to discuss this condition with the client. Which of these facts must the nurse have knowledge of?
    a. Endometriosis increases the risk for spontaneous abortions.
    b. Endometrial tissue is typically found in the uterus and around the ovaries.
    c. Endometrial tissue causes more problems in the second trimester.
    d. Endometriosis increases the risk for a low fertility rate.
163. A first-time mother asks about the need to be checked for gonorrhea between 6 to 8 weeks. What is the best response by the nurse?
    a. There is a need to find out to be prepared for altered growth and development of the fetus.
    b. Early detection allows for better treatment during the pregnancy.
    c. Gonorrhea may cause abnormalities to the baby in utero.
    d. Gonorrhea is passively transmitted through the placenta.
164. A home health nurse is assigned to the following clients. In planning the visits for the day, which client would the nurse schedule as the first stop?
    a. A 4-day postoperative client
    b. A mother 3 days post-delivery with a need for newborn care instruction
    c. A client diagnosed yesterday with diabetes that requires insulin injections
    d. A client who has decubiti that require dressing changes
165. In which of the following situations is a toddler at highest risk for lead poisoning?
    a. The toddler chews on lead pencils.
    b. The toddler lives next door to old apartments.
    c. The family of the toddler lives in an old house.
    d. The daycare center where the toddler visits three times a week is located in a historic building.

Answers, Rationales, and Test Tips

1. The correct answer is c.

Rationales
    a. Hyper-jaundiced sclera is a finding of clients with terminal liver

failure from cirrhosis, hepatitis, or other chronic liver problems.

b. Flapping tremors occur from elevated serum ammonia levels when the liver fails. They may be documented as an asterixis.

c. Irritability is commonly found at the onset of the delirium tremens sequela.

d. Seizure activity more likely happens in the terminal stage of delirium tremens.

Test Tips

Key words in the question are "In addition to confusion and visual hallucinations." This pinpoints what the question is asking about, the initial stage of delirium tremens. Key words in the options are irritability and flapping. Irritability tends to be associated with the initial findings of hypoxia or elevated toxins. The word flapping depicts a type of tremor that is consistent with liver failure, not liver dysfunction. No information in the stem indicates "liver failure." For this situation the time frame is critical. The beginning of the time line for delirium tremens, not the end of the time line where seizure activity occurs, is being questioned.

2. The correct answer is b.

Rationales

a. The gag reflex usually returns a few hours after endoscopic procedures. This situation is not in that category of time.

b. Initially a decrease in oxygen leads to irritability, anxiety, agitation, and hostility or to an increased level of consciousness.

c. Dehiscence is from poor wound healing and typically occurs a week or two after surgery. As indicated in the stem, this client's situation is probably within the first 3 to 4 days after surgery. It is too soon for separation of the incision.

d. If a client had difficulty in swallowing, the swelling in the neck would be greater than just "slight." Think anatomy: the esophagus is behind the trachea. Thus the airway is most likely to be compromised first.

Test Tips

Key words in the stem give clues for the nurse to look for findings of a lack of oxygen. These are: "after radical neck," "feeling of swelling in the neck area," "the drainage system is . . . patent," "evaluate for . . . anticipated findings," which means initial findings. If you had no idea of the correct answer, try giving themes to each option such as: option a, GI; option b, neurologic or oxygenation; option c, healing; option d, GI. It is obvious that option b would be a priority over the other options. Do not confuse difficulty swallowing with difficulty in breathing. One can have severe difficulty swallowing without an impingement in the upper respiratory tract. For example, a person with a sore throat has difficulty swallowing but no significant impairment of breathing.

Time in this situation is another important factor to guide your approach for critical thinking. The gag reflex returns within a few hours after endoscopic procedures. An increased level of consciousness is an initial finding associated with a lack of oxygen or glucose to the brain. With a feeling of swelling in the neck, a client might be experiencing pressure on the trachea resulting in a narrowed airway. Dehiscence is a separation of an incision usually within 7 to 14 days after surgery. It occurs from poor healing associated with conditions such as diabetes, obesity, malnutrition, and steroid use. Severe difficulty in swallowing would be associated with more severe findings other than what is given in the stem ("feeling of swelling"). The drainage system would probably be sluggish or blocked.

3. The correct answer is b.

Rationales

    a. This question is more likely associated with a self-esteem problem. This question might be asked during a follow-up session but not in an acute situation when the client exhibits a severe condition.

    b. This question is more likely associated with withdrawn behavior. More often depressed clients are withdrawn and act isolated rather than being active and outgoing.

    c. This question might be asked later in the therapy of a depressed client or a client who has attempted suicide. The feeling of hopelessness, sometimes from a perception of an inability to have some control over events, may further a client's depression. To respond to this open-ended question may be an overwhelming task for a client with a severe depressive disorder. Recall that severely depressed persons exhibit minimal verbalization and movement.

    d. This question might be used if a client was admitted for an acute psychiatric condition other than depression or if the client was being counseled at a mental health crisis center.

Test Tips

The type of option will sometimes help you to select the best answer. Let's review these.

Options a and b are yes or no questions; options c and d are open-ended questions. Option d sounds good until you recall that the client has "severe depressive disorder." Recall that depressed clients commonly do not talk or move much. At this time, upon admission and the initial interview, the yes or no question format is better than open-ended questions for this type of client. Note that in general open-ended questions are better to use with most clients. Exceptions to this rule of thumb are clients who suffer from acute depression, mild to severe respiratory distress, cognitive impairment, or a history of being a "rambling historian" (for example, clients who, if asked about chest pain, start to tell about chest pains experienced 10 years ago).

4. The correct answer is d.

Rationales

    a. This option is too general to be the best answer for most multiple-choice questions.

b. A temperature of 102 is of concern for any client, whether an adult or a pediatric client. However, without other information in this particular stem, this option is too narrow and specific to be the best choice.

c. This information indicates a neurologic deficit from a lack of circulation to brain tissue on the opposite side from the weak side. The hypoxic tissue might occur from a lodged clot, a leaking vessel, or sickled cells. This is a complication of, not a reason for, sickling.

d. This information describes a situation that might result in severe dehydration, which could initiate a sickle cell crisis. Other causes of crisis are severe infection, hemorrhage, and, sometimes, high levels of physiologic or psychological stress.

Test Tips

The first step is to identify what the question is asking. The client should identify which of these findings is a reason for sickling to occur. The complications of the sickling process have nothing to do with this question.

Other clues lie in the key words of the options. In option a, "some" describes an unknown amount. In option b, a T 102 without other findings is given. In option c, "weakening . . . one side" indicates stroke-like findings, which can be complications of the sickling process. In option d, "severe . . . thirst" indicates severe dehydration which can initiate the sickling process. The reason for sickling, not the complications of sickling, is what is asked for in this question. Don't get stuck on the words "loss of blood" in option a. The amount of blood loss is important, however, in most questions.

5. The correct answer is b.

Rationales

a. Placenta previa occurs from the low implantation of a placenta. The bleeding is typically bright red and of small to larger amounts depending on the location of the implantation over the uterine opening. Treatment is either strict bed rest for the mother or a cesarean section if the placenta separation and bleeding is significant. Predisposing factors include decreased vascularity of the upper uterine segment, multiparity, use of cocaine, and scarring from prior surgeries.

b. Abruptio placenta occurs as a premature separation of a normally implanted placenta from the wall of the uterus. The blood is typically a darker red. Treatment is usually an emergency cesarean section. Predisposing factors include fibrin defects, pregnancy-induced hypertension, use of cocaine, older multigravidas, and involvement in motor vehicle accidents.

c. A ruptured uterus, a rare occurrence, is more likely to happen from some type of trauma situation.

d. This answer, "a fetal incident," is a nondescript type of statement. It is probably not a good choice for the answer to any question.

Test Tips

Go with what you know. Focus on the key words "abdominal pain." Avoid reading into this as "cramping" or "contractions." Focus on the fact that abdominal pain at 36 weeks is not typically normal. Avoid clouding your thinking by getting stuck on the word "exquisite." Exquisite means fierce, excruciating, severe, or harsh.

If you haven't heard about PPP, now listen up: Bleeding associated with **P**lacenta **P**revia is **P**ainless. In option b, associate that anything abrupt usually results in emotional or physical pain. Associate a crisis as being abrupt. No data is given in the stem to support a ruptured uterus. Option d is too general to be correct. Be cautious not to read this as a "fatal" incident.

A last clue is the time frame of the episode, which directs you towards thinking of this as a one time event. The 36 weeks gestation, third trimester, narrows the options to a or b since abruptio placentae and problems associated with placenta previa commonly occur then.

6. The correct answer is b.

Rationales

a. Eliminate this option since no information is given to require a repeat of the lab test, especially without a physician's order.

b. Since the lab results suggest a significant decrease in renal function over the past 3 days, the client's neurologic state, especially the level of consciousness, and the electrolyte potassium levels are essential to consider at this time.

c. Vital signs and the ECG report are correct items to further assess. However, these are not the best actions since vital signs are a more general evaluation of overall body function and the ECG is more specific to cardiac changes than renal changes. In this situation, the kidney is the focus. Thus an option with specific renal-related evaluations would be better.

d. The initial part of this option is correct as a first action. The second part of this option is not specific to the evaluation of renal function. A heart rate and rhythm may be only indirectly impacted by renal failure. Acute changes to high levels of potassium may affect the heart's function.

Test Tips

Use the approach of pretending to take a report in order to increase clarity of thought in deciding about first actions. Of the data, note that creatinine levels went from 2 to 5 in 3 days. Report the actions in the options: option a, repeat lab and notify MD; option b, ✓neuro and ✓K; option c, VS and ECG report from AM; and option d, ✓LOC and monitor HR for rate/irregularity.

Then look for lab or data clues in the

options. For option a no information is given to support the repetition of this lab test. If the information stated that there was great difficulty getting the blood sample with a possibility of hemolyzed blood, then new blood would need to be drawn. Hemolyzed blood typically will result in higher serum values. Option b supports the use of the nursing process, to do further assessment prior to intervening. In option c, "take vital signs" sounds good but it is too general for this specific question. Asking for an ECG report directs one to look for changes in the waveforms from high serum levels of electrolytes, specifically potassium or magnesium. These are usually elevated in renal failure. Option d, the verb "check" is okay but to "monitor" is not the best answer for a question that asks for "first actions." There is no time element to the "monitoring" and therefore this is not the best answer.

7. The correct answer is c.

Rationales

a. Nausea is an initial finding for digoxin toxicity in adults. In infants it is manifested by poor feeding since infants cannot communicate feelings of nausea. Vomiting may accompany nausea when adults become digoxin toxic.

b. The change to a decreased level of consciousness in infants is more reflective of drops in oxygen or glucose, or of dehydration or infection.

c. Poor feeding indicates that an infant has no appetite or has anorexia. Typically an infant has to eat before vomiting. Thus vomiting would usually not be an early finding of toxicity in infants. Infants, unable to communicate with words, can only communicate to the caretaker by refusal to take the bottle or by taking less formula.

d. A racing heart is too general an option to be the best answer. An infant's heart can race with minimal stimulation such as during the change of a diaper.

Test Tips

It is crucial to note that the client is an infant. See prior discussion of each option under Rationales above. The onset of toxicity is a clue that directs you to think of initial findings.

8. The correct answer is a.

Rationales

a. In acute asthma events three findings occur: an increase in thick secretions, an inflammation of the mucosa of the lung, and a narrowing of the bronchioles. For the administration of an antiinflammatory to be most effective, the bronchioles need to be dilated.

b. In maintenance therapy for clients with asthma, clients may be advised to take the antiinflammatory first and then the bronchodilator. Recall that with maintenance therapy the bronchioles would not usually be constricted.

c. This is too general an option to be the best answer. Avoid reading into this option and misperceiving it to say "inhalation treatments with a mist."

d. This option has little to do with the "sequence" of therapy. As written it is an isolated action.

Test Tips

The key words in the stem, "best sequence" and "acute . . . event," give you clues to focus on what is critical to a person who can't breathe. Think physiology: the airways need to be opened first. Therefore option a is the best answer.

9. The correct answer is d.

Rationales

a. The increase in productivity and liquidity of pulmonary secretions is the effect of the mucolytic, Mucomyst, or may simply be from an increased intake of water and other fluids.

b. A decrease in the frequency of coughing results from the ingestion of an antitussive or cough suppressant. Cough syrup with codeine is one of the more common combinations prescribed.

c. In option c the sustained increase in a heart rate is an expected effect from bronchodilators such as aminophylline. If the heart rate exceeds 120 beats per minute the nurse should report this to the physician.

d. The feeling of nervousness is a common side effect of bronchodilators. Sometimes the physician may decrease the dosage of medication if the nervousness bothers the client. The twitching of a client's muscles is representative of possible theophylline toxicity.

Test Tips

The key words in the stem are "expected reportable effects." Think in terms of what findings require notifying the physician. *Recall tip:* The major drug classification of aminophylline is bronchodilator. Bronchodilators are typically given by aerosol for a faster action in acute respiratory distress. However, aminophylline is unable to be given by aerosol, and so is given by IV at slow rates. It takes 2 to 4 hours to get the blood levels up to where this medication is effective. Therefore it is usually started simultaneously with aerosol bronchodilators.

10. The correct answer is b.

Rationales

Options a, c, and d are correct statements. The statement in option b requires the nurse to clarify that the B_{12} injections are given every month. Bimonthly means to give the injections every 2 months.

Test Tips

Key words in the stem include "a need . . . to clarify." After reading the question, you should approach the options to look for the one that is an incorrect statement. Read all of the options. Avoid reading so fast as to misread option a, selecting it and not reading the remaining options. As you look for the key words in the options, note the small words. In option a, "no" can be easily overlooked, resulting in a misreading of the statement. In option b, "bimonthly" might be read as monthly and therefore not selected. In option d, "no longer" may be misinterpreted as an absolute and not chosen because of the rule that it's best not to select options with absolutes. Beware: selecting or not selecting an option because of one rule is the wrong approach.

11. The correct answer is b.

Rationales
All options—Note that all of the vegetables (except the potatoes) are foods included in the high vitamin K group, green leafy vegetables. Of these three vegetables, the greens are the greenest in color and therefore have the most vitamin K. Vitamin K interferes with the action of Coumadin on the clotting system.

Test Tips
Recall tip: The antidote for too much Coumadin, as measured by a prolonged prothrombin time (PT >1½ or 2 times normal), is an injection of vitamin K. The effects of Coumadin continue for 7 to 10 days after it is stopped. Just to review, if the dosage of Coumadin is increased, it will take 48 to 72 hours to see the full effect of the change, an increase in the PT.

If you are unsure of the correct answer, an approach to use is to cluster three of the options under the vegetable group "green leafy." Then identify which would be the most detrimental for this client to eat (i.e., which has the most vitamin K).

The client is currently on an oral anticoagulant. Keep in mind that the prothrombin time is most likely regulated by the client's usual diet. Lab values may change if excessive foods with vitamin K are consumed. If the anticoagulant had been stopped that day or earlier, then the selection of food type is no longer a priority.

12. The correct answer is a.

Rationales
a. Kidney beans are high in vitamin B_6, pyridoxine, which helps to prevent or to control peripheral neuropathies. Peripheral neuropathies are an expected side effect of the antitubercular medication. In contrast, kidney beans and other legumes that are high in pyridoxine are to be avoided when a client with Parkinson's disease is on dopamine agents. Pyridoxine inhibits the action of dopamine agents.

b. Steamed broccoli is classified as a green leafy vegetable. Green leafy vegetables are high in vitamins C and K. This vegetable would not be contraindicated in clients treated for tuberculosis. It may help in the healing of the lung tissues.

c. Aged cheeses have no associated significance in the treatment of clients on these medications. Aged cheeses, which contain tyramine, are to be avoided in clients being treated with a MAO inhibitor, an antidepressant.

d. Baked fish has no associated significance in the treatment of clients on these medications. Baked fish may be suggested for someone on a weight loss, low-cholesterol, or low-fat diet.

Test Tips

A clue in the stem is the statement that the client is taking multiple medications. Recall that only a few conditions have therapy with multiple drugs over long periods of time. These are tuberculosis (6 to 18 months), antineoplastic therapy (6 to 12 weeks), AIDS (time varies), asthma (for life), and certain cardiac conditions such as hypertension or angina (for life).

Remember to go with what you know. Option b is associated with vitamin K and anticoagulants. Option c is associated with the antidepressant group, MAO inhibitors. Eliminate these options, then choose between options a and d. Using common sense and the knowledge that baked fish is usually a safe choice of food in any condition, select option a.

13. The correct answer is b.

Rationales

a. Avoid misreading the question to think it is asking about an interference with the absorption of the medication. If you do, you will select this option, Tums antacid, as the correct answer. Recall that Tums are high in calcium.

b. Potato chips are high in sodium and carbohydrates. This excess salt intake usually results in the excess elimination of lithium through the kidneys. Therefore the therapeutic levels of lithium are decreased. The client may exhibit an increase in manic behaviors.

c. Bananas are high in potassium and fiber. They are good for potassium replacement and preventing constipation.

d. Chocolate chip cookies are high in sugar and the chocolate has cocoa, which is a stimulant. Both might contribute to more manic behavior. Neither will affect the serum levels of lithium. Recall that the client is on Lithobid, a mood stabilizer which helps to modulate manic behaviors.

Test Tips

A key word in the stem is the name of the medication, Lithobid. Associate "lith" with lithium, used for clients with bipolar disease to control the degree of mania. Recall that lithium is often considered as lithium salts and is sensitive to serum sodium levels. The other key words are "taken in excess." So think excess salt.

As you read the options, use associations to clarify your thinking: Tums, calcium; potato chips, salt; bananas, potassium; chocolate, cocoa. Simply match salt concerns in the stem to the option with salt—option b. Use this approach only if you have no idea of the correct answer.

14. The correct answer is b.

Rationales

   a. This statement is not a true statement. Insulin needs are based on other factors such as exercise and emotions in addition to diet. If the sympathetic system is stimulated, glucose is increased in the blood as a normal physiologic response. Emotions such as happiness, sadness, anger, and fear can trigger a sympathetic response.

   b. This statement describes Type I diabetes mellitus. These clients are required to get insulin injections. In Type II diabetes mellitus, the beta cells slow their production of insulin. Therefore clients with Type II can take oral hypoglycemics, which stimulate the beta cells to produce more insulin.

   c. This option might be considered as a correct answer, especially if you read into it to think that nonfunctional means no insulin production. However, identify that the statement is too general to be the best answer. Also, scarring may not be the cause for a lack of insulin production in all cases of Type I diabetes mellitus.

   d. This is a false statement about Type I diabetes mellitus. There is no "progressive" decrease in pancreatic function as associated with insulin production and Type I diabetes mellitus.

Test Tips

The key words in the stem are "most accurate" and "Type I." Refer to the rationales above. In option c, the word "nonfunctional" is accurate and the word "scarred" is inaccurate since the cause of the failure of insulin production is sometimes unknown. In option d the statement "progressive decrease in pancreatic function" is false for a Type I diabetic. This statement might apply to Type II diabetes.

The time reference "some days . . . needs are minimal" in option a leads you to think of insulin coverage with blood sugar checks. Beware. In this approach you have introduced information into the option and the overall situation. The time given with the information "as you get older" in option d is correct information for a Type II diabetic. But be alert: the question is about Type I diabetics.

15. The correct answer is a.

Rationales

   a. Since oral medications go through the liver, they have an opportunity to damage the liver. Some medications are more toxic to the liver than others and result in liver damage with elevated liver enzymes. In contrast, some medications, because of a hepatic first-pass effect, are inactivated by the liver enzymes before the drug reaches the systemic circulation. Note the key words "oral . . . agents" in the stem.

b. Renal function is more commonly affected by agents given IV rather than oral agents. Creatinine level, normally around 1, is monitored for elevation, which occurs with renal damage.

c. Cardiac enzymes have no association with oral chelating agents, which are given for lead toxicity. Cardiac enzymes are monitored for increases with coronary artery spasms or occlusions. They are CK-MB and LDH.

d. Pancreatic enzymes are not influenced by oral chelating agents. These enzymes are monitored for increases with acute or chronic pancreatitis. They are amylase and lipase.

Test Tips

If you are unsure of the correct answer, here's how to make an educated guess. Eliminate options c and d, cardiac and pancreatic enzymes. They are typically affected by damage to the organ from lack of oxygen or trauma. Think of the normal digestive process and that oral agents are detoxified or changed in some manner in the liver and then move to the kidneys for excretion. Note the clue in the stem: "transient changes," not "permanent changes." This approach guides you to select liver enzymes.

16. The correct answer is a.

Rationales

a. These are the most common terms used to describe the action of different types of insulin. An easy way to recall the sequence is to compare drawing up insulin to the characteristics of bath water during a bath. Bath water is clear when the bath begins and gets cloudy as the bath continues. Short acting insulin, a clear liquid, is drawn up before intermediate insulin, a cloudy liquid. Short acting insulin is described as regular insulin or Humulin R. Intermediate acting insulin is described as NPH or isophane insulin suspension or Humulin N.

b. This is an incorrect sequence.

c. Short acting is an appropriate description of insulin. Extended acting is an inappropriate description for insulin types.

d. Regular acting is an uncommon way to describe insulin.

Test Tips

Go with what you know as you read the options. Try reading the options in a vertical manner as you think of "the most recommended sequence." The word "sequence" suggests for you to look for a first then a second action. This will help you to narrow the options to two more quickly. The most common ways to label the insulin types are short and intermediate acting. Narrow the options to a and b. Reread the question and the first part of each option.

Another way to recall the correct sequence is to associate that short acting insulin is a liquid one can see through; short acting insulin is regular insulin. The intermediate insulin is NPH, which you cannot see through. Draw up clear, then cloudy. A final way to recall the correct sequence is to associate RN, registered nurse, with Regular first then NPH second.

17. The correct answer is b.

Rationales
  a. This is a correct position for IM injections. However, mannitol is not given IM. It is typically given by IV drip or IV push.
  b. This is a correct action and the best answer. The question is focused on the prevention of complications.
  c. This is a correct action. It is not the best option since taking blood pressures is not an action aimed at the prevention of complications. Taking blood pressures may result in the identification of a complication. Also this option is quite narrow since other factors such as HR or RR may also be monitored and the monitoring would typically last throughout the administration of the medication, not just for 1 hour.
  d. This option is a correct action when mannitol is given. Also, the action of this drug results in an increased urine output since it is an osmotic diuretic. This option has a focus of evaluation of medication effectiveness, not complication prevention.

Test Tips
Key words in the stem, "during mannitol administration . . . to prevent complications" help you focus on complications

during administration. Options b, c, and d are correct actions. Note, however, that option b has the use of a filter for prevention. If you had no idea of a correct answer, simply match the key word in the stem, prevention, with the option that contains the key word. Remember that the question usually holds the clues to the selection of the best option.

The time of "during" administration is also important to note as you read the question. The time frames of before, during, and after are essential to identify the correct option. In option d, to "monitor blood pressure every 15 minutes for 1 hour" is too restrictive and incomplete. More commonly assessments are made every 15 minutes × 1 hour, every 30 minutes × 2 hours and every hour × 4. Remember that the frequency of these is adjusted based on the evaluation of the desired outcome.

18. The correct answer is a.

Rationales
  a. This is the correct dosage. *Recall tip:* There are **60 M**in. in **1 Hr.** Associate this with the conversion of mg to gr.: **60 Mg** in **1 Gr.** Thus ¼ Gr would be obtained by dividing 4 into 60, which is 15 mg. At this point reread the question to identify what dosage is ordered and when it is ordered to be given. Then select the correct answer.
  b. This is an incorrect dosage.
  c. This is an inappropriate action. Medications are sent from a pharmacy in the form available at an agency.

d. This is an incorrect action. There is no information given in the stem to suggest the medication is needed in a liquid form. Just because it states a child is receiving it is no reason to get a liquid form. If the client in the stem was an infant or neonate, then obtaining the medication in a liquid form would be the best action.

Test Tips

The required dosage versus the available form and dosage are important factors to identify. The type of medication and the fact that the client is a child are irrelevant to answering this question. Avoid focusing on the wrong item, a child, and then reading into the option that the child cannot swallow a pill and needs a liquid form of the medication. Beware that your personal experience or biases can cause you to add information to situations given in test questions.

During the reading of the first part of options c and d you may have introduced your own thoughts into the second part of these options. On this type of question, attempt first to calculate the correct dosage from the given information before reading the options. The medication is ordered "BID" which is twice a day.

19. The correct answer is b.

Rationales

a. The dose is not excessive. Penicillins are commonly ordered in dosages of a million units.

b. Since penicillin injections are usually 4 to 5 ml per injection site and given deep (Z track) injection, the nurse needs to explore the client's experience with prior injections. These injection sites are commonly sore for a few days. This information needs to be collected at the onset of the client-nurse interaction, before the client is positioned and the injection is given.

c. This is a true statement. This action would follow the action in option b, once the nurse gained more information.

d. This option is half correct. The nurse should check for allergies—but to penicillin, not sulfa.

Test Tips

Key words in the stem, "action . . . at the onset of the client-nurse interaction," help you to think in terms of a sequence of actions. The verbs in the options—discuss, inform, or ask—help you focus on a sequence of action. Usually the normal sequence before drug administration is to ask, discuss, and inform. Asking about allergies to medications, foods, or contact agents is a priority. Note what allergy is given in the option in relation to the medication given in the question. A common error is to focus your thoughts on the initial part of an option instead of carefully reading the second part of an option. In this case, an allergy to sulfa has nothing to do with penicillin. Next the nurse usually discusses any concerns of the client. The final action is for the nurse to inform the client of the requirements of the client during the process of drug administration.

A final clue is given in the time frame: "at the onset of the client-nurse interaction." It sets up the picture for what the nurse would do first upon entering the room and approaching the bedside.

20. The correct answer is a.

Rationales

   a. Ipecac syrup, an emetic, elicits the therapeutic response of vomiting by the stimulation of the chemoreceptor trigger zone along with an irritation of the stomach. Follow the 5 to 15 ml of syrup with 200 to 300 ml of water to enhance the effects. Bouncing the child after administration may increase the emetic effect. Vomiting is to be avoided when caustic substances are ingested.

   b. Milk may be given to neutralize the caustic hydrocarbons.

   c. Oxygen administration is a supportive action for the respiratory system. The threat to the lungs from aspiration is greater than the threat to the gastrointestinal tract or the systemic effects, which are generally mild. Observe the child's increased respiratory effort and congested lung sounds, which are indications of pneumonitis.

   d. Intravenous antibiotics are part of acceptable therapy that is given for prophylaxis to prevent pneumonia or as treatment for it.

Test Tips

Key words in the stem are "ingestion of hydrocarbons." Identify that these are petroleum-based substances such as gasoline, kerosene, and turpentine. An immediate concern after ingestion of these substances is aspiration, which can cause severe chemical pneumonitis. Other key words are "plans to question." Be careful. Avoid misreading the question as asking what would the nurse plan to do instead of "plan to question".

If you are not sure of the correct answer, give each option a theme—emetic, fluid, oxygen, antibiotic. Sometimes identification of the given drug's classification will clear your thinking. Another approach is to go with what you know based on the general treatment of any problem. Cluster three of the options with the focus on general treatment. Fluids, oxygen, and antibiotics are commonly given for a general treatment or the prevention of complications. Therefore the emetic given for specific treatment is probably the correct item to question on the physician orders.

21. The correct answer is d.

Rationales

   a. You may have narrowed the options to a and d. You are on the right track. Liver tenderness is a finding with an enlarged liver, which can be a result of the Tylenol overdose. It could be a complication. However, keep in mind that liver tenderness is a subjective assessment since the practitioner determines the degree of tenderness. Therefore with the other given objective assessment factor in option d, an elevated serum enzyme level, liver tenderness is not the best option.

b. A decreased ALT, a liver enzyme, indicates the liver is healing.

c. As it is stated, this option is too vague to be the best option. Recall that therapeutic levels of prothrombin are 1½ to 2 times normal. However, remember that this client had an overdose and is not on oral anticoagulants.

d. Further elevation of enzymes after an initial insult to an organ indicates further damage and complications. This is true for the enzymes of the heart, the liver, and the pancreas. Note that this is the best answer since the measurement of serum levels is an objective assessment.

Test Tips

Avoid misreading the question to think that it is asking about findings of Tylenol overdose instead of the complications. "Decreasing" serum levels 6 days after ingestion of Tylenol is a desired effect for evaluation that therapy is working. Avoid misreading decreasing as increasing. In option c, "slightly sustained . . . elevated" are vague words that give no definition to the actual measurement of prothrombin time. In option d, "further elevation" indicates that the levels are increased from the initial elevation. Note that therapy for a client with a Tylenol

overdose usually lasts 4 to 5 days with Mucomyst given orally. At 6 days post therapy the liver enzymes should be near normal if complications are absent. No specific lab values are given in this question or in the options. The concept of enzyme elevation is crucial. When an organ is damaged the enzymes for that organ elevate; as healing occurs the enzymes will fall back to within the normal range. Continued or increased elevation indicates sustained or increased damage.

22. The correct answer is a.

Rationales

a. With the overuse of laxatives or enemas, the intestinal tract becomes dependent upon an external stimulation. This results in minimal spontaneous peristalsis.

b. This is an incorrect answer. Thinning of the intestinal mucosa is not a result of laxatives. Chronic use of some medications such as steroids may result in a thinning and easy bruising of the skin not the intestine.

c. Identify that Epsom salts is under the major drug classification of a laxative. Recall that laxatives stimulate the large intestine. This option is about the stomach, the wrong anatomical location to best answer the question. An imbalance of acid in the stomach is also more likely to be an intermittent problem than a continuous physiological problem.

d. This is an incorrect answer. Recall that absorption especially of proteins mainly occurs in the small intestine, not the large intestine. Laxatives stimulate peristalsis. Increased peristalsis does little to alter the absorption process of nutrients. However, it does decrease the time available for the nutrients' exposure to the intestinal wall.

Test Tips

"Major physiological" helps you to think of what normal physiology has changed as you read the options. "Epsom salts" or magnesium citrate falls under the major classification of a laxative. Laxatives stimulate peristalsis. You may have been looking in the options for dehydration or fluid/electrolyte loss. Note that option d has "altered absorption," but of protein-like nutrients. As you read the key words in option a, recall that "spontaneous . . . peristalsis" means by itself, without external stimulation. In option c, "stomach" provides a clue. But it is the wrong anatomical location, since laxatives act mainly on the intestines and not on the stomach.

23. The correct answer is d.

Rationales

a. Anemia is a more common finding in heroin addicts since the craving for the drug is greater than the craving to eat. Therefore these clients usually eat little and are at risk for anemia.

b. The offer of sexual favors in exchange for money or drugs is a frequent behavior pattern in heroin addicts. Sexually transmitted diseases such as syphilis may be found.

c. IV drug abusers are a high-incidence population for tuberculosis from poor living conditions and nutritional deprivation.

d. Symptomatic bacteremia is more likely to be an acute condition. The client would more likely come to a health care facility because of high fever, fatigue, and other findings of a systemic infection. Screening is least likely for this infection.

Test Tips

The words "least likely screened" are critical to note in the stem. If you read too fast, you will misread the question and select the most likely problem. Then you will have greater difficulty selecting d, the best option, because options a, b, and c are associated with heroin use. In situations such as this, the best approach is to return to the question, reread it, and attempt to reword it. As you reword the question your error in reading will become evident.

If you have little idea of the correct answer, the use of a theme for each option will help you decide what option to choose. Think of chronic versus acute conditions. Anemia is a chronic condition; syphilis and tuberculosis are both insidious and potentially chronic types of infectious diseases. Symptomatic bacteremia is an acute condition. Think of heroin use as a chronic addiction. Contrasting the options as acute or chronic may help your recall of information. Cluster the three similar options associated with chronicity and subtle findings, options a, b and c. Select option d, the odd man out.

24. The correct answer is d.

Rationales

a. Osteoarthritis, a chronic local joint problem, is often treated with moderate to high doses of aspirin when clients have pain. Typically the pain occurs intermittently with an increase in humidity or with overuse of the affected joint.

b. Coronary artery disease is treated with low doses of aspirin, 65 or 81 mg per day.

c. Rheumatoid arthritis, a chronic systemic disease, is often treated with high doses of aspirin, 2000 to 5000 mg per day in divided doses, in acute exacerbations. However, the treatment is commonly intermittent since the disease has periods of remission.

d. Lupus erythematosus, a generalized connective tissue disorder, is treated with steroids and/or nonsteroidal antiinflammatory drugs, of which aspirin is a common choice. The dosage is usually high, 2000 to 5000 mg per day, and given in divided doses. This is the best answer since clients with this disease take higher doses more continuously and for longer periods than clients with the diseases given in the other options.

Test Tips

"Priority" of instruction is a clue that all of the options will be correct answers. Keep this in mind as you read the options. Avoid the approach of looking for three incorrect options if the question is asking for a priority, the first, or an initial something.

What do you think of when all of the given diseases are of a chronic nature? You think of treatment: Is it intermittent or continuous in nature? Then you think of the medication in the question: Does it have different strengths of doses for different diseases?

25. The correct answer is b.

Rationales

a. This is correct information to give the client. It is not the best response of the nurse since it does not give any details.

b. This is the best response by the nurse since it gives the most detail and answers the client's question about "why" there is a need to continue the medication.

c. This statement is not accurate information to give the client. It also does not answer the client's question of "why."

d. The information in this option is partially true. With diet and exercise changes and the loss of weight some clients can come off of their antihypertensives. However, note that the stated diet is very low sodium; this is incorrect information. This option does not answer the client's question of "why."

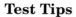

Test Tips

The key words in the stem, "why is there a need," give you a specific focus to look for when you read the options for the nurse's best response.

In option a, "a lower level" is a vague answer for a specific client question. In option b, the specific information of "within normal ranges" for the blood pressure and the other specific information about the organs gives the client specific information for the specific question that was asked. The initial part of option c is correct but the conclusion, to be weaned off the medication, is incorrect. Besides, not all antihypertensives require a weaning off period of 2 to 5 days. Some are just stopped when a different medication is prescribed. Option d answers a client question of "when can I come off" of the medicine. In addition, the words "very low" are distractors. They are commonly misread as "low" or "little." Option d is often read too quickly since it is the last in the series of options.

26. The correct answer is a.

Rationales

a. A precipitous delivery, one that is fast, does not allow time for the fetal head to mold as it travels the birth canal. Thus the result is trauma to the fetal brain.

b. Uterine stimulation, a result of Pitocin effects, may end in uterine tetany, which is given in option c. This option b is too general of an option to be the best answer since it does not specify the degree of uterine stimulation.

c. With tetany of the uterus the fetus most likely becomes hypoxic. Damage occurs to the fetus, but it is not fetal "trauma."

d. Water intoxication is a complication of the administration of Pitocin. Findings may include a severe increase in blood pressure, severe headache, visual disturbances, and edema. The effect on the fetus would be hypoxia.

Test Tips

The question being asked is this: "Fetal trauma" is the result of which effect of the drug Pitocin? If you read too quickly you probably came up with a different question; that makes option selection more difficult. Reading the question more slowly a second time will help you find your error of missing key words like "fetal trauma."

Did you identify that all of the options are effects of Pitocin? Did you then go back to reread the question? Options b, c, and d can be clustered under the umbrella of "the end result is fetal hypoxia." Option a, standing alone, is the odd man out. Select option a.

Another approach is to ask: Is the time frame fast or slow? Of the given options, option a occurs fast and cannot be repeated, as can the other options. A fast time frame without repetition is typical of any kind of trauma. Note that the question is asking about fetal trauma. Make the association between the fast time, no repetition, and trauma to select option a.

27. The correct answer is d.

Rationales

a. Vasopressin, an antidiuretic hormone (ADH), is under the general drug classification of a pituitary hormone. It is used to treat diabetes insipidus and postoperative abdominal distention. It promotes reabsorption of water by action on the renal tubular epithelium. It also causes vasoconstriction and is used in events of bleeding esophageal varices. Available forms are nasal spray, cotton pledgets, or IM/SC. The form Pitressin Tannate is given IM/SC every 2 to 3 days for chronic therapy.

b. Tapazole, under the general drug classification of an antithyroid hormone, is given for hyperthyroidism, thyroid surgery preparation, and thyrotoxic crisis. It inhibits the synthesis of thyroid hormones by decreasing iodine use in the manufacture of thyroglobulin and iodothyronine. It does not affect already formed hormones. Clinical responses in about 3 weeks include increased weight, decreased pulse and blood pressure to within normal ranges, and decreased T_4.

c. Protropin, a pituitary hormone, has the action of growth hormone. It is given to treat dwarfism in children. It is usually given IM.

d. Decadron, a corticosteroid in glucocorticoid classification, is used to treat inflammation, allergies, cerebral edema, septic shock, collagen disorders, and some neoplasms. It can be given IV, IM, or PO. This medication requires weaning to prevent adrenal crisis.

Test Tips

The name of the drug is important. If you have no idea of the correct answer, you could compare the drug names. Note that the drug in the stem ends in "sone." Now look the options. The drug in option d ends in "sone." Simply match the endings, since the question is asking about the same instruction for two drugs.

Recall tip: **T**apazole **T**reats **T**hyroid that is **T**oo active. *Identification tip:* Drugs ending in "tropin" can be associated with growth hormone, and drugs ending in "sone" usually fall under the classification of steroids.

28. The correct answer is a.

Rationales

a. Ticlid, a platelet aggregation inhibitor given by mouth, has been found to reduce the risk of strokes in high-risk clients. If the client is on long-term therapy, blood studies such as prothrombin time and CBC and liver and kidney function studies need to be monitored. Advise clients to avoid the use of aspirin while on this drug, since both act in a similar manner.

b. Streptokinase, a thrombolytic enzyme, dissolves clots. It is used in acute clinical situations such as acute myocardial and cerebral infarction. Administration is by IV pump in emergency or critical care units. This drug falls into the advanced care category and is more likely an incorrect answer if found on a basic nursing exam.

c. Heparin, an anticoagulant, is given in higher doses for acute embolic situations to prevent further clot formation, and in lower doses for prevention of thrombus in situations where clients are on bed rest or are minimally active. Recall that heparin, which is only given IV or SC, requires administration by a licensed person.

d. Amicar, a hemostatic, inhibits fibrinolysis and therefore stabilizes a clot. It is used for situations of cerebral bleeding from leaky aneurisms. Administration is by IV pump in critical care units. This drug falls into the advanced care category and is more likely an incorrect answer if found on a basic nursing exam.

Test Tips

In the stem, "to prevent further pathology" gives you the action of the drug to look for in the options. The first thing to do as you read the options is to place each drug in a major drug classification. By doing so, you can eliminate options b and d. Refer to the discussion above under Rationales. Next think of the route of each of the drugs. Heparin you know is IV or SC; Ticlid you may not even know since this may be a new drug name

for you. Go with what you know. The question is asking in *general* about prevention of clots and not about an *acute* situation. Therefore eliminate the heparin and select Ticlid.

29. The correct answer is b.

Rationales

a. These are lab tests that are specific to the clotting factors that are produced in the liver. They are not the best answer since they measure only one part of liver function. The best option is the test that looks at the overall function of the liver.

b. These lab tests are indicators of overall liver function. Therefore they are the best choice to answer the question. Recall that most PO medications require filtering through the liver. Thus if labs need to be monitored, it is usually the liver tests. ALT is the old SGPT and AST is the old SGOT.

c. LDH or lactate dehydrogenase is an isoenzyme found in many tissues. Alkaline phosphate is found in highest amounts in the liver, biliary tract, and the bone. Therefore this is not the best option since the given tests are not specific to the liver.

d. Ammonia levels are specific to a liver that is in failure, not just dysfunction. When liver function fails, ammonia is not converted to urea, which is normally then excreted via the kidneys. Thus ammonia levels rise and BUN may fall. The high ammonia levels irritate the nerve endings. The result is the classic finding of asterixis— a bilateral flapping tremor of the hands. AST is a test for general liver function. Refer to the discussion under option b.

Test Tips

You do not have to know what this drug classification is to answer the question correctly. Approach the options knowing that the client is on a PO medication for a long time—over a period of months. Think of what you know and try to apply it to the given question. What other drugs are given for a long time? A most common classification is antitubercular drugs for tuberculosis. At this point you may have had your memory jogged and thought of the liver enzymes. Go with what you know.

As you read the options, look for groups of tests that are specific to one organ. Eliminate option d since these tests could relate to many places in the body. Of the remaining options, think of specific versus general liver function. The tests in option a measure a specific function; in option b, a general function; and in option c, a combination of general and specific. Go with option b, tests for general liver function.

"Every few months" for lab testing indicates that the client will be on the medication for many months or perhaps continuously. The individual levels of the lab tests are not important by themselves. However, patterns of changes such as increases from the normal range are of concern and indicate organ malfunction. As the organ heals, or the medication is stopped or decreased in strength or frequency, the values will typically decrease towards the normal range.

30. The correct answer is d.

Rationales

a. Valium, a centrally acting muscle relaxant, has the side effects of drowsiness, dizziness, bradypnea, hypotension, and flaccid muscles.
b. Soma, a centrally acting muscle relaxant, has the side effects of drowsiness, dizziness, bradypnea, hypotension, and flaccid muscles.
c. Flexeril, a centrally acting muscle relaxant, has the side effects of drowsiness, dizziness, bradypnea, hypotension, and flaccid muscles.
d. Dantrium, a peripherally acting muscle relaxant, works directly on the skeletal muscles. It decreases the availability of calcium in the muscle and thereby decreases the contractility of the muscles. Its primary use is to decrease spasticity of the muscles in chronic conditions such as multiple sclerosis, cerebral palsy, spinal cord injuries, and strokes.

Test Tips

In the stem, the words "directly relax" are a clue that the selected drug will not have any central nervous system effects. If you are not sure of the correct answer, go with what you know and use a cluster technique. Cluster Valium, Soma, and Flexeril under the classification of muscle relaxants that make clients drowsy and sleepy. Select the odd man out, Dantrium, a drug that you probably never studied in school.

31. The correct answer is b.

Rationales
  a. Cogentin, an anticholinergic agent or cholinergic blocker, is given to minimize the Parkinson's disease-like findings or extrapyramidal (EP) effects associated with the neuroleptic drugs. Antipsychotic agents are also called neuroleptics. Vitamin B_6 has no interaction with this drug.
  b. Rifampin, an antitubercular agent, is given over a 6- to 18-month period for tuberculosis. A major side effect is neuritis from the inflammation of peripheral nerves from a B_6 deficiency. Giving the vitamin helps prevent the neuritis.
  c. Levodopa, an antiparkinsonism drug, helps to relieve the symptoms of the disease. It does not cure the disease. Vitamin B_6 *interferes* with the drug's *effectiveness* and therefore vitamin supplements of B_6 need to be avoided or foods high in vitamin B_6 need to be restricted. Foods high in B_6 are lentils, oatmeal, walnuts, beef kidney and liver, bran products, yeast, and avocados.
  d. Prostigmin, an antimyasthenic agent, is given to clients with myasthenia gravis, a chronic condition of

fatigue and weakness of the voluntary muscles. These agents do not cure the disease; they help the clients maintain a normal lifestyle. Vitamin B_6 has no effects on the drugs. Antimyasthenic agents are also used to reverse the effects of neuromuscular blocking agents. Normal levels of potassium are needed to have the best effect from antimyasthenic agents. The antidote for too much antimyasthenic agent is atropine sulfate.

Test Tips
In the stem, the words "protect the nervous system" are clues that guide you to think as you read the options: which drug causes nervous system side effects? As you read each option, give each drug a major classification (refer to the Rationales above). Then think of a few major side effects for each drug classification.

32. The correct answer is c.

Rationales
  a. Antianxiety agents have effects on the central nervous system. Some common side effects are sedation, orthostatic hypotension, abuse, dependence, and tolerance.
  b. Antiparkinsonian drugs relieve the extrapyramidal *symptoms of the disease*. They do not have extrapyramidal side effects.
  c. Antipsychotic agents, also called neuroleptics, have as a major side effect serious movement disorders. These include extrapyramidal effects such as tremors, tar-

dive dyskinesia (involuntary rhythmic movements of the face, limbs, or trunk), dystonia, impaired muscle tone, and akathisia (restlessness, agitation, an inability to sit still).

d. Psychotropic is an umbrella term for the drug classifications of antipsychotics, antianxiety agents, antidepressants, and mood stabilizers.

Test Tips

In the stem, "the addition of" is a clue that the given agents will have the side effect of extrapyramidal effects. If you misread the question to ask about extrapyramidal effects in general, then you probably selected option b as you thought of Parkinson's disease. If you narrowed the options to c and d, remember to go with what you know. You know you have studied antipsychotics. If you are unfamiliar with the word psychotropics, and cannot recall anything specific, then go with what you know and select antipsychotics.

33. The correct answer is c.

Rationales

a. Catecholamines include norepinephrine, epinephrine, and dopamine. These have the action to vasoconstrict. The end result is hypertension, not hypotension.

b. Histamine response is a result of the body having an allergic reaction to some antigen. Think of sinus allergies to pollen or dust. The nasal passages become congested from the histamine response, which causes local vasodilation and congestion. Or think of the bee sting site; it becomes swollen from the histamine response of vasodilation. In major allergic reactions like anaphylaxis the client will exhibit hypotension or shock. However, note that none of this information has anything to do with this question about a consequence of spinal anesthesia.

c. If the sympathetic system is blocked, the vessels are unable to constrict to maintain blood pressure. Therefore there will be hypotension. This is the consequence of spinal anesthesia. The blood becomes pooled in the lower torso; preload is decreased to the right heart and the blood pressure drops.

d. Parasympathetic blockade results in findings of sympathetic effects—hypertension, tachycardia, tachypnea, dry mouth, and pallor. Recall that the parasympathetic system modulates the bodily functions to maintain the day-to-day processes of digestion and elimination. Thus the mouth is moist; the respiratory and cardiac function is controlled within normal ranges for rate and function; and the peristalsis of the bowel and bladder results in normal patterns of elimination.

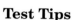

Test Tips

Hypotension leads you to think of the vasodilation of the vessels as a result of medication administration in the form of spinal anesthesia. If you have no idea what a catecholamine is, then do not select this as your answer unless you know the other options are incorrect. Associate histamine with an allergic response, the most common of which is sinus allergies. Be careful. You may have misread option c as sympathetic "effects" since you were thinking of effects that cause hypotension. Again, in option d, be careful not to misread this as parasympathetic "effects." If you did, you probably selected this as your answer. For parasympathetic blockade effects think of the effects of atropine HCl.

34. The correct answer is c.

Rationales

a. This seems like a good answer at first glance. However, upon a second reading, "a resting position" seems too general of a statement. The fact that the client has an acute head injury takes precedent. Recall that the goal is to prevent further increases in intracranial pressure, so the head of the bed usually needs to be elevated at least 10 to 15 degrees.

b. This is a correct action for this client. However, it does not best answer the question in regard to the time (right after completion of the admission assessment).

c. This is the best action upon completion of the admission assessment. Such activities include placing the head in alignment, creating a quiet environment, dimming the lights, and elevating the head of the bed at least 10 to 15 degrees.

d. This is a correct action for this client. However, it does not answer the question in regard to the time (right after completion of the admission assessment).

Test Tips

Key words in the stem help to clarify your thinking. "Upon completion . . . the admission" provides the important time frame clue. "Most indicated" helps to prepare you that all of the options are appropriate interventions (correct). Your approach is to decide which one has the highest priority. "Acute" guides you to think of concern about increases in intracranial pressure. In contrast, a "chronic" head injury client has priorities for mobility and communication.

Key words in the options further your ability to use critical thinking. In option a, "resting position" is a vague description for positioning. Since the client has had an acute head injury, the head of the bed must be kept up a minimum of 10 to 15 degrees and the head kept in alignment. If the client did not have an acute head injury this would be the best answer. In option d, "prevent constipation" is an action for any client admitted to an acute care facility. For any client, being on bed rest decreases peristalsis and increases the risk of constipation. If you missed the time frame, you probably chose this option.

35. The correct answer is d.

Rationales
  a. This is an incorrect statement. Arteriogram procedures do not include the removal of the dye. The dye is removed after an oil-based myelogram is completed via a spinal tap or lumbar puncture.
  b. The first part of this statement is true. The second part is incorrect information.
  c. This is incorrect information for the procedure of a femoral arteriogram. Regional anesthesia is done for arm, hand, pelvic, or lower extremities surgery. It is sometimes done when the risks of general anesthesia are too great.
  d. This is a correct statement. Local anesthesia is sometimes used for the insertion of an arterial catheter or line in the radial artery.

Test Tips
The key word in the stem, "arteriogram," provides the location for the needle insertion. Recall that arteries are tough, thick vessels and are sometimes difficult to cannulate. Pressure and pain may result if no anesthesia is used.

Be careful with two-part options. The tendency is to read the first part carefully and skim over the second part, especially if the first part is a correct finding. If you have this error pattern and select a two-part option, reread it with the second part first before making a final option selection. In option b, "nausea at the time of injection" is correct. "Nausea the remainder of the day" is incorrect information. Both options c and d are similar except for the type of anesthesia. If you have no idea of the correct answer, use your common sense. For a needle stick into an artery it is more reasonable to numb the area locally than an entire region of the body. Select option d.

Recall tip: As background information, it is important to note that a femoral arteriogram is an x-ray procedure where dye is injected into an artery. Any dye injected into the body acts as a diuretic and clients will have an increased urine output after the procedure for about 24 hours. Therefore a nursing action postprocedure is to force fluids unless contraindicated by other given medical conditions.

36. The correct answer is b.

Rationales
  a. This is a good choice, but not the best choice of the given options. Be cautious not to have chosen this option based on what you may have seen in your clinical experience.
  b. This is the best answer. Walking shoes provide for the best support and gripping during walking on a treadmill.
  c. Clean socks have nothing to do with the support of the feet while walking.

d. Covering the shoes is not a concern during a stress test, which is not done in a sterile environment.

Test Tips

The key words in the stem, "stress test," give you the clue that the client will be walking at a fast pace during the test. "During the test" clues you in to select an item that will stay on and support the feet. The words "12-lead ECG stress test" help you to focus that the heart will be monitored as the client walks at various paces and elevations of the treadmill.

In the options, "sturdy" may have distracted you into thinking of slippers that are like shoes. The bottom of this type of slipper may be appropriate, but slippers are just that—easy to slip on and off. They would be a threat to safety if used for walking at a fast pace on a treadmill.

37. The correct answer is b.

Rationales

a. Aspirin is a nonnarcotic analgesic, which would be appropriate for mild pain. However, note that the client has bone marrow suppression since the client has to receive Neupogen. Thus it is reasonable to conclude that the client's platelets are also likely to be low. Clients with bone marrow suppression should avoid drugs like aspirin that decrease platelet aggregation and increase the risk of bleeding.

b. Acetaminophen, also a nonnarcotic analgesic, is the better choice of drug for this client.

c. A narcotic analgesic is not the best choice of pain medication when the pain characteristics are not actually given, or the type of cancer or the length of time the client had the cancer is not described in the stem.

d. A narcotic analgesic is not the best choice of pain medication when the pain characteristics are not actually given, or the type of cancer, or the length of time the client had the cancer is not described in the stem.

Test Tips

In the stem, the absence of the description of the cancer or the length of time the client had the cancer (Is it in the end stages?) is a clue to go with the less extreme option or less potent medication. If you have no idea of this medication, associate "neu" with neutrophils, a type of white blood cell in the body. Remember, the red and white blood cells are formed in the bone marrow. So if this medication is given, it logically follows that the bone marrow is being stimulated to produce white cells. Furthermore if the bone marrow is forced to work, bone pain may result. In fact, the most common side effect of Neupogen is bone pain. This type of pain is readily relieved by nonnarcotic analgesics.

Another approach to determining the

best option is to identify the drug classification of each of the medications. Eliminate the strongest medications, narcotics (options c and d), since no specific information is given on the pain severity. Of the remaining choices, eliminate aspirin since it has multiple effects on the body (of which bleeding is the most severe).

38. The correct answer is a.

Rationales

a. The central venous pressure, CVP, is the indicator of the preload of the heart. Preload is the volume of blood returned to the heart. Therefore it is a reflection of the total volume pumped *through* the heart.

b. Peripheral arterial pressure is the pressure of the blood *after it leaves* the heart. It is measured invasively by an arterial line or noninvasively by cuff blood pressures.

c. Pulse oximeter readings have nothing to do with the volume of blood through the heart. It is a noninvasive measurement of arterial oxygen saturation, normal being a minimum of 90% and a maximum of 100%. For accurate readings, clients need normal hemoglobin and hematocrit, warm fingers, toes or earlobes, and systolic blood pressures of at least 90.

d. The heart rate will increase with too much volume or too little volume traveling through the heart. It is not a good measurement of the volume pumped through the heart.

Test Tips

In the stem, "effectiveness of . . . Lasix" tells you to look for volume changes in the circulation. Recall preload is volume associated with blood return to the heart and afterload is resistance associated with blood leaving the heart. Preload is measured by CVP, neck vein distention at a 45-degree head elevation, or pulmonary artery pressures. Afterload is measured by arterial blood pressure. Also in the stem, "reflection of total volume pumped through the heart" gives the location of concern. Of these words, the word "volume" further defines what to look for in the options—one that has to do with volume. Read all options and then reread them with the intent to identify the one that deals with volume. Refer to the Rationales.

39. The correct answer is d.

Rationales

a. Lethargy and sleepiness are findings of glucose levels that are too high. Think of glucose as the fuel to the brain: when it has too much, it gets lazy and wants to sleep (maybe just like you, when you have too much to eat).

b. Agitation is an initial finding with a drop in blood sugar from a maintenance level. However, coordination of motor skills is a normal finding and has no implication in a change of glucose levels.

c. Confusion may be an initial finding with a drop in glucose levels. However, insomnia is an inappropriate finding. The question has the time frame of 2 hours, not 24 hours.

d. Restlessness and irritability are classic findings of a drop in or a low glucose level.

Test Tips

The first action is to identify that the IV solution is a hypertonic solution because of the high glucose, usually a 10% solution for peripheral and a 20% to 25% solution for central hyperalimentation. The second action is to note that the time parameter of "within the initial 2 hours of infiltration" is an important time for the glucose to drastically drop since the solution is no longer running. Therefore in the options you will be looking for findings of hypoglycemia.

Your approach to reading a series of items within each option should not be to read the options with a single thought. Use the vertical reading process. Read only the first item in each option: lethargy (eliminate immediately since it is a finding with hyperglycemia), agitation, confusion, and restlessness. Remember that you're looking for findings of hypoglycemia in reading the second item in each option: coordination of motor skills (eliminate this since it is a normal finding) and insomnia (eliminate this since it usually has nothing to do with glucose levels). So option d is the only one left and is the correct answer.

40. The correct answer is b.

Rationales

a. Keeping NPO before the exam is incorrect advice for this client. Clients are kept NPO for 12 to 14 hours before most invasive tests or procedures.

b. This is the correct information—omit stimulants to the brain for at least 24 hours prior to the test for the prevention of hyperactive brain waves. Other substances to avoid are sodas, chocolate, and tobacco products. Clients are advised to omit substances that would also slow the brain's activity.

c. Withholding drugs prior to tests is done only with a physician's order. Sometimes these tests may be done to evaluate the effectiveness of a drug.

d. The initial part of this option is correct if the client is on anticonvulsants. The second part of the option is incorrect. A lack of glucose to the brain from not eating or drinking actually increases brain activity.

Test Tips

"Electroencephalogram" is a noninvasive test of the brain's wave activity for seizures or hyperactivity or a slowing. The client must have clean hair and scalp. Small electrodes with a paste are placed in the scalp for the test. Post care is to ensure the hair gets washed for the comfort of the client.

The first option is a distractor since

many invasive tests require being NPO. If you chose this option and didn't read the other options, be aware that you have a higher risk of failing exams. If you read the other options only superficially and still chose option a, you also are in a high-risk category for doing poorly on exams. When you think option a is the best answer before you've read the other options, the action to take is to simply stop. Go to option d and read it; then read option c; then read option b; and, lastly, read option a again. Reading the options in a backward sequence increases your attention to detail. It is a matter of mentally processing the given information, and this is helped by reading the options in reverse order.

41. The correct answer is c.

Rationales

a. "Risk for" is a potential diagnosis. In this given situation an actual nursing diagnosis is more appropriate since the question is asking for a "priority."

b. This is an actual diagnosis and sounds good. However, no information is given to support findings of poor nutrition. Having diarrhea would not be an indication of poor nutrition. Findings of poor nutrition might be thinning hair, emaciation, and enlarged abdomen. Think of the pictures of starving children. Besides, nutrition is not a priority at this time.

c. Fluid volume deficit is a priority since the circulation is affected by a lack of volume. This is a more immediate and severe threat to the client than the other nursing diagnoses given.

d. Skin impairment is not a priority for this client even though the client is immunosuppressed. The circulation factors are more important and are validated by the data of "constant dizziness when initially standing." Besides, there is no information in the stem to validate skin impairment. Having diarrhea does not validate skin breakdown.

Test Tips

The given clinical findings assist you to validate the nursing diagnoses. Only options b, c, and d are validated by these. However, persistent diarrhea and muscle cramps are indirect indicators of altered nutrition. Both of these findings suggest there might be a potassium deficit. Keep in mind than "nutrition" has a broader connotation than just an electrolyte imbalance. Dizziness when initially standing is a classic finding with fluid volume deficits such as dehydration from constant diarrhea.

As you read the options, first identify the actual and potential diagnoses. Since the question asks for the priority, the actual diagnoses in options b, c, and d are better choices. Then compare the diagnoses with the given clinical findings to validate them. Options b and c remain after this step. Then if you are having trouble deciding, put a theme of the organ system to each: option b is gastrointestinal (GI) for nutrition; option c is cardiovascular for circulation of fluid. Select option c since cardiovascular concerns have a priority over GI.

42. The correct answer is c.

Rationales

a. This is a true statement. Usually when clients with TB no longer cough, they are considered non-contagious.

b. This is a true statement. Since the child has multi–drug-resistant TB, therapy typically takes place over longer periods of time than with TB.

c. This is an incorrect statement. You may have missed it because you simply failed to read carefully the second part of the option. The use of a tissue is appropriate since it is disposed of after use. However, a handkerchief is usually kept in a pocket and used over and over again. Therefore there is a risk of spreading the bacillus to others from the dirty hanky that harbors the organism.

d. This is a true statement. These foods have higher amounts of vitamin B_6, which helps to prevent the peripheral neuropathies, a side effect of antitubercular medications.

Test Tips

Note that the tuberculosis is "multi–drug-resistant." Therefore therapy is usually needed for longer periods of time than with other tuberculosis. "A need for further teaching" guides you to look for an incorrect statement. As you read the options, note and be wary of two-part options. Take care to read the second part carefully; or, read it first and the first part second.

43. The correct answer is a.

Rationales

a. This is the correct action of Reglan, a cholinergic drug that stimulates the gastrointestinal tract. It helps to tighten the esophageal sphincter for the prevention of gastric reflux into the lower esophagus. Reflux of gastric contents is the more common cause of esophagitis.

b. The first part of option b is a correct statement about Reglan. However, if you did not read carefully, you would not have identified that this drug does not have antiinflammatory properties.

c. The first part of option c is a correct statement about Reglan. However, Reglan does not stimulate gastric secretions. Food and fluids entering the stomach stimulate the release of gastric secretions.

d. The drug that protects the gastric mucosa is Carafate. This requires it be taken on an empty stomach.

Test Tips

"Esophagitis" helps you to locate where the problem is. If you have no idea of a correct answer, simply match the anatomical location in the stem with the same from an option (option a). All the other options have the anatomical location of the stomach ("gastric").

If you chose options b or c, make a note if it was because you did not carefully read the second part of the option. If this is so, from here on out make it a routine that on two-part options you will read the second part first and the first part second. This will help you to make more accurate and correct decisions.

44. The correct answer is b.

Rationales

a. Lithium levels are important to monitor. However, with these clients clinical findings are of equal importance. Therefore this is not the most dangerous action of the client.

b. Lack of sufficient salt in the body increases the risk for lithium toxicity. Recall that lithium, a salt, attaches to sodium and is excreted via the kidneys. So with little salt in the body there is less lithium excreted. The result may be lithium toxicity. Clients who sweat a lot are also at risk for toxicity.

c. With increased sodium from sodas the client will most likely have an increased excretion of lithium with the sodium. Thus the therapeutic level of lithium will be down and the client might manifest more manic behaviors. This isn't as dangerous for the client as possible toxicity.

d. Lithium has a category D rating for pregnancies. Definite fetal risks are possible; it may be given in spite of the risks if needed for life-threatening conditions. Lithium crosses the placenta and does enter the breast milk.

Test Tips

The key words in the stem, "which action . . . is most dangerous," help you to take the approach that all of the options are dangerous. Your task is to decide which is the "most dangerous." Therefore as you read the options, do not look for an incorrect action.

As you read the options, condense each of them into a few words to help you with your critical thinking skills. Option a, lithium levels every other month; option b, little salt in diet; option c, lots of salt in diet; and option d, pregnancy concerns in the future. Of these options, a and c can be eliminated as most dangerous since they don't affect the client on a daily basis. Of the options left, remember that too little salt is more dangerous for this client because of the risk of toxicity.

45. The correct answer is c.

Rationales

a. This is a correct option but is too general to be the best answer for this question.

b. This is an incorrect action. Water-soluble, not oil-based lubricants are used to facilitate passage of tubes into any orifice of the body.

c. This is a correct action. The problem is with catheter insertion, and this approach—to have the client participate—helps in the learning process.

d. This statement is incorrect since glycerine suppositories result in stimulation of the intestine and not in moistening of the mucosa.

Test Tips

Identification of the problem—insertion of the catheter—helps you to narrow the options to b or c. Then go with what you know: water-soluble lubricants are more commonly used. Select option c.

If, however, you have no idea of the correct answer, make an educated guess to narrow the options to b or c since the client is active in the procedure. Option d states to "suggest to the client" so this is not an action that will solve the client problem now. The time frame suggests that action be taken while the problem occurs.

46. The correct answer is a.

Rationales

a. These findings are most suggestive of medication interactions. These are adverse effects associated with lithium toxicity. Enalapril, an antihypertensive in the ACE inhibitor group, increases lithium levels when taken concomitantly.

b. These are general findings of middle-aged females who may be entering the perimenopausal stage of life.

c. Slight kyphosis has nothing to do with drug interactions. It is an age-related finding in women who lack appropriate calcium levels. The other two findings are noted among middle-aged females who may be entering the perimenopausal stage of life.

d. The first two findings are suggestive of findings of middle-aged females who may be entering the perimenopausal stage of life. Sleepiness is a nonspecific finding that could be associated with many factors.

Test Tips

If you are not sure of the correct answer, simply approach the options with the evaluation: Is the finding normal for this client's age (a middle-aged female) and normal for drugs in general? You may have no idea of what these drugs are. Use the vertical technique to read the series of items in the options for a clearer approach. *Recent* memory loss is not considered normal for the age or for drug effects in general. A borderline BP, kyphosis, and feelings of panic and anxiety fall into the category of normal for age. Even though at this point you are pretty sure that option a is the best answer, continue to read vertically each item in the options. Upon completion of this reading sequence it is evident the muscle weakness and hyperreflexia are abnormal findings. Thus they are most suggestive of medication interaction.

Recall tip: Other than in lithium toxicity, hyperreflexia is found in preeclampsia and eclampsia from the low magnesium levels. Thus magnesium drips are given and the client's deep tendon reflexes and ankle clonus are checked to determine and monitor the amount of magnesium given to the client.

47. The correct answer is b.

Rationales

   a. This is considered a noninvasive test and there is no need to restrict food or fluids. Electromyography (EMG) aids in the diagnosis of muscular dystrophy, amyotrophic lateral sclerosis (ALS), and myasthenia gravis by evaluating electrical potential associated with skeletal muscle contraction.

   b. Valium is to be omitted along with any other muscle relaxants, since they cause a loss of muscle tonicity.

   c. They may experience some discomfort from the needle insertion into the muscles. However, this option indicates negligible discomfort.

   d. Clients may have to move their muscles voluntarily during the procedure. Lying still is incorrect data for this test.

Test Tips

A first step is to identify the type of test. If you have no idea, simply break the word apart: electro = electricity, myo = muscle, ography = to examine. Thus this is a test to measure the electrical current to and from muscles. If you have no idea of a correct answer, read your options and go with what you know. You probably are sure about options a, c, and d. In option b you recall that the drug classification for Valium is a muscle relaxant. Make an educated guess or just match muscle test in the stem with the option that refers to muscle, option b.

In option c, "very little or no pain" is not realistic for any procedure. Usually any diagnostic test has some degree of discomfort even if it is just lying on a hard, cold, x-ray table.

Recall tip: Tests that allow clients to eat or drink are ECG, EEG, and EMG. The "E" means the client usually can eat and drink. With the EEG, foods or fluids that contain stimulants need to be withheld at least 24 hours prior to the exam.

48. The correct answer is d.

Rationales

   a. The actions in this statement are incorrect.

   b. The actions in this statement are incorrect.

   c. The actions in this statement are incorrect.

   d. This is the proper method of disposing of a narcotic analgesic.

Test Tips

"Narcotic analgesic" is a clue that actions need to be different. Use a true or false approach to each option as you read through them. From how the question is stated, there is only one correct answer.

49. The correct answer is c.

Rationales

a. This is incorrect information. Other antineoplastics might be given to enhance the effect of one another.

b. Antiemetics are given prior to treatment to decrease the side effects of nausea.

c. Recall that chemotherapy drugs for cancer cause increase catabolism with the rapid destruction of the cancer and some normal cells. Anti-gout medications such as allopurinol (Zyloprim) reduce endogenous uric acid by inhibiting the action of xanthine oxidase.

d. This is incorrect information. Folic acid conversion is a distractor since it sounds good.

Test Tips

The key words in the stem, "anti-gout medication," help to guide you to option c with the word gout in it. If you are not sure of the correct answer, match the key word(s) in the stem with the same word(s) in an option.

50. The correct answer is b.

Rationales

a. Anticholinergics are not given to prevent nausea. Antiemetics are given to prevent nausea in some situations.

b. Anticholinergics (of which atropine is the most common) are given to prevent bradycardia. The action of anticholinergics is to speed up the heart rate and increase the electrical impulse conduction through the heart.

c. Urinary retention is a side effect of anticholinergics since they decrease peristalsis of the bowel and the bladder.

d. Anticholinergics have no effect on respiratory depression.

Test Tips

The key words in the stem, "purpose of prevention," assist you to think of the ABCS (airway, breathing, circulation, and safety). So you could narrow the options to b or d since these are the most serious problems given in the options. Use your knowledge plus common sense to note that the stem tells you what the action of anticholinergics is on the respiratory system. The next system, therefore, is the cardiac. So select option b, cardiac arrhythmia.

Another approach is to give each option a theme: option a, GI; option b, cardiac; option c, urinary; option d, respiratory. The stem already has addressed the respiratory; select the cardiac option since the urinary and GI systems are of less importance.

51. The correct answer is c.

Rationales

a. Antacids, such as Mylanta and Maalox, neutralize stomach acid.

b. Carafate is the medication that protects stomach mucosa by coating it. It has to be taken on an empty stomach.

c. This is the primary effect of histamine H_2 receptor blocking agents. These agents include Tagamet, Zantac, and Pepcid.
d. Cholinergics such as Reglan increase gastric peristalsis.

Test Tips

The key words in the stem, "primary effects," guide you to look for the major action of these drugs. Beware that if you are used to saying "H_2 blockers" you may not have recognized this drug group. In preparation for any exam be sure to review and know what the most common abbreviations mean.

Recall tip: The words gastric and stomach are interchangeable. The intestine begins after the pyloric valve, which prevents intestinal contents from returning to the stomach. When there is a small bowel obstruction, the fluids back up into the stomach and clients typically have bile-colored emesis.

52. The correct answer is d.

Rationales

a. Erythromycin, an antibiotic, has a bactericidal action rather than a bacteriostatic action. Bactericidal agents result in the killing of bacteria. In contrast, something with bacteriostatic action tends to restrain the development or the reproduction of bacteria.
b. There is no difference in the absorption rate since both of the given medications are ointments.

c. There is no difference in administration since both of the given medications are ointments.
d. Erythromycin is less irritating to the eye than the silver nitrate ointment, which may also discolor the skin (this is called argyria). Tetracycline and erythromycin are given in most agencies because they not only treat gonococcus but chlamydia infections as well.

Test Tips

Both medications are ointments: so options a, b, and c can be eliminated since there is only minimal difference in their absorption rates, administration techniques, and lasting effects. Eye ointment is usually given for local application rather than systemic effects, so eliminate option b. Bacteriostatic effects are usually found in the soaps that adults use to decrease the number of bacteria on the skin and decrease body odor from sweating. Most antibiotics have a bactericidal effect.

53. The correct answer is c.

Rationales

a. This may be an appropriate action but it is not a priority. Also note that the client is a child of 6 years of age. To keep a young child in a 30-degree elevation would be difficult. This degree of elevation is more appropriate with adults who are post cardiac catheterization.
b. Blood pressure checks are appropriate but not the priority after this procedure.

c. This is the priority after a cardiac catheterization for a client of any age. In children sometimes a cutdown is done rather than a blind stick so there is less risk of bleeding from the cutdown site. The quality of the pulse needs to be compared between the right and the left extremities. An absent or weakened pulse may indicate arteriospasm or an occlusion of the vessel.

d. Coughing forcefully is to be avoided since it results in the Valsalva maneuver, which stimulates the vagus nerve and slows the heart.

Test Tips

The age of the client guides you to be cautious as you read the options. "Priority action" allows you to anticipate that all of the options are correct actions and you need to identify the sequence of actions. In option d, "cough forcefully" is inappropriate after any type of cardiac procedure. It is appropriate after pulmonary diagnostic tests. The first few hours are critical for monitoring the pulses, since this is the time when complications are most likely.

54. The correct answer is d.

Rationales

a. This action is important to teach since the child may not take all of the food or fluid after the medication is mixed with it. Also remember that, for developmental reasons, the toddler has picky eating habits.

b. Remember the age of the client. This is appropriate information for the parents. Heart rates less than 100 could indicate digoxin toxicity.

c. These clinical findings might suggest digoxin toxicity. This information is important to teach.

d. Since this is a child and the medication is digoxin, the physician's office should be called for advisement if a dose is missed. Note that the digoxin is ordered two times a day, not once a day as adults usually take it.

Test Tips

The key words in the stem, "least desirable," are essential. They are the clue for you, as you read the options, to list them in order of priority. The correct answer here is the one on the bottom of the list. Options b and c remind you that the client is a child. The remaining options could distract you into thinking "adult," since there is no reminder of a child. This confusion as you read might happen if you are extremely tired or tense.

55. The correct answer is a.

Rationales

a. Hematuria indicates active bleeding and needs to be reported. The therapy may need to be adjusted or the client may need clotting factors enhanced. This would be based on the severity of the hematuria.

b. Isolated premature ventricular contractions are expected effects from either the myocardial infarction or the thrombolytic therapy.

c. This change is a good change. It shows that therapy is effective and the heart does not have to work as hard.

d. An increase in pain relief is a desired result of the therapy. There is no need to notify the physician before rounds.

Test Tips

"Thrombolytic and anticoagulant therapies" are the clues to choosing option a. Before regularly scheduled rounds indicates that it is urgent to notify the physician.

56. The correct answer is d.

Rationales

a. Calcium is needed for clients in middle age and especially elderly women, pregnant women, and clients with healing bones.

b. Foods high in iron are recommended for clients with anemia and for pregnant women.

c. Foods high in protein are encouraged for clients with trauma, postsurgical or other, who have increased healing needs.

d. Thiazide drugs are potassium-depleting diuretics. Magnesium loss often accompanies the potassium loss with these diuretics.

Test Tips

Associate thiazide diuretics with the loop diuretics that result in potassium loss via the renal tubules. If potassium isn't an available answer, look for another electrolyte. In this case you have to choose between calcium and magnesium. Go with what you know: calcium loss is not commonly associated with diuretic use, so select magnesium.

57. The correct answer is c.

Rationales

a. This may be a normal finding for a 2-year-old child with or without nephrotic syndrome.

b. These are expected findings in children with nephrotic syndrome.

c. A nasal discharge in itself is not a concern. However, the cloudy nature is an indicator of infection. Children with nephrotic syndrome are very susceptible to infection because of treatment with corticosteroids, the loss of proteins, and their generalized edema, which makes the skin more fragile and susceptible to trauma. Prompt treatment is essential as with any client who is immunosuppressed.

d. This is an expected finding in children with nephrotic syndrome.

Test Tips

Identify nephrotic syndrome as a chronic condition, and with any chronic condition there is some degree of chronic stress with resultant immunosuppression. The other key phrase in the stem to guide your selection of an option is "most concerned." This lets you know that all of the options are correct and that you have to prioritize them and select the first on the list.

"Cloudy discharge" is a consistent warning that infection is present. If the drainage is whitish, it is more likely to be associated with an allergy.

58. The correct answer is b.

Rationales

    a. Weighing is not required for either of these two medications. Observing for skin changes and possible allergies is important for either of these medications. But because of the weighing, this is not the best answer.

    b. Fluids are crucial when sulfonamides are given, to promote their excretion and to prevent crystalluria and kidney stone formation. In addition, if the client has a severe infection that requires two antibiotics, then the client is probably dehydrated from a high temperature. It is important to rehydrate the client to keep the kidneys functioning.

    c. Blood pressures are more appropriate if clients are on cardiovascular or diuretic medications, not antibiotics.

    d. These findings are of a concern but not with these two types of medications. Hyperreflexia might occur if there is low magnesium from a medication such as a diuretic. Be careful not to confuse photophobia (sensitivity of the eyes to light) with photosensitivity (sensitivity of the skin to sunlight).

Test Tips

If you have no idea of a correct answer, note that the medications given are general classifications rather than specific names of drugs. Therefore a more general option would be the best. Options a, b, and d have more specific items in them, so they probably aren't the best choice.

    Another approach is to find a theme in each of the options: option a, nutrition/skin; option b, renal; option c, circulation; and option d, neuro. When antibiotics are administered, the renal system is most important for the excretion of the dead bacterial waste products and the metabolized medication.

59. The correct answer is a.

Rationales

    a. Severe back pain on one side may indicate acute renal calculi or gallbladder attack. In this situation the client was on a sulfa drug for over a week. If fluids were not forced, crystals from the sulfa drug may have caused the formation of kidney stones. There is no information given to suggest a problem with the gallbladder.

    b. This option leads you to think that the client has possibly had this pain before taking the medication and now it has increased in frequency. Also the information is general in that it does not state what the pain is associated with as in option c, which is more specific.

c. Even though this pain is severe, it is associated with eating. So it isn't the best option to answer the question about this medication.
d. This finding may be a normal finding for this client, who is elderly.

Test Tips
The sulfa drug Azulfidine is a clue to possible complications of renal origin. Even if you did not know this, go with the other key words "priority concern" and select option a that has severe pain. Caution: even though option c has the word severe in it, the pain is associated with eating. So it is not the best choice for the answer.

60. The correct answer is c.

Rationales
a. This is an incorrect action (to use a large syringe and aspirate gastric contents). When gastric contents are aspirated and not returned to the stomach, the client may go into a metabolic alkalosis from the loss of acid.
b. These are incorrect actions.
c. This is the best action of the given options. With infants, a much smaller amount of air is inserted to check the tube's placement.
d. These are incorrect actions.

Test Tips
If you are not sure of the correct answer, go with what you know. The client is a newborn, so everything will be not just smaller but very small. After reading the options, identify that option c is the most similar to the procedure for adults. Therefore make an educated guess; it is probably the best answer.

61. The correct answer is b.

Rationales
a. Only anticonvulsants can directly delay seizure activity. Mannitol might delay seizure activity indirectly by decreasing brain swelling and thus prevent tissue irritability.
b. This is a correct action of mannitol, since it is an osmotic diuretic. It pulls fluid from tissue and interstitial spaces.
c. Catecholamines such as epinephrine constrict the cerebral arteries. Other substances such as tobacco products, caffeine, and chocolate will also constrict arteries and veins.
d. Antiinflammatories such as steroids decrease inflammation. Some of these used for brain injury are Solu-Cortef, Solu-Medrol, and Decadron.

Test Tips
Read each of the options to give each a general drug classification. Refer to Rationales. Think physiologically: when there is bleeding, there is swelling. To decrease the swelling, fluid must be pulled from the site or arterial constriction occur to prevent further blood accumulation. This is why you ice an injury for 24 hours, then apply heat after 24 hours.

62. The correct answer is a.

Rationales

   a. Think virus. Chickenpox is from a virus and so is herpes zoster, which is better known as shingles. Shingles can be very painful and can occur anywhere on the body. Once a person has chickenpox, the virus is ever-present in a dormant state in the body. Stress and other factors can result in a flare-up.

   b. Canker sores, ulcerous lesions in the mouth, are not associated with the chickenpox virus.

   c. This has nothing to do with nerve involvement of the face.

   d. This information introduces new information and is not correct.

Test Tips

If you have no idea of a correct answer, group the options b, c, and d under the types of questions the nurse would ask *before* the client had been diagnosed. Since the client has a diagnosis of herpes zoster, a more specific question about exposure to a virus is the best answer.

63. The correct answer is d.

Rationales

   a. Ultrasonography is usually noninvasive and not painful. No reason exists to give sedation.

   b. No iodine injection is given with this exam. For an IV cholangiogram, dye is injected and this would be an appropriate question.

   c. Before invasive procedures clients are kept NPO for 8 to 12 hours.

   d. This is the best answer. The nurse would explain that the noninvasive test is to examine the gallbladder for gallstones or enlargement. The procedure includes the use of conductive gel (which will be cold) and a probe that will be moved around the right upper quadrant of the abdomen.

Test Tips

If you have no idea of what this test is, use a cluster technique on the options. Cluster options a, b, and c under the umbrella of specific information about a procedure. Option d, the general information, is the odd man out and the correct answer.

64. The correct answer is d.

Rationales

   a. Histamine H_2 receptor blocking agents inhibit the secretion of hydrochloric acid into the stomach.

   b. The breakdown of protein is done by pepsin in the stomach and peptidases and pancreatic secretions in the small intestine.

   c. If the client had the problem of gastric ulcers, then this would be the correct answer.

   d. In renal failure the antacids Amphojel and Basaljel are given to bind the phosphate in the intestines and be excreted in the stool. Kayexalate, an exchange resin, is given PO or by enema to bind the potassium in the intestine and be excreted in the stool.

Test Tips

The clue is in the stem—the client has chronic renal failure. Now review the options for one or two words that describe what that option is about: option a, hydrochloric acid; option b, proteins; option c, gastric secretions; and option d, phosphate. Recall that the focus is renal failure. The only option that can be associated with renal failure is option d. Recall that in renal failure there are increased serum levels of potassium and phosphate.

65. The correct answer is c.

Rationales

a. Repositioning the client is more appropriate for mild to moderate pain.
b. Giving a back rub is more appropriate for mild to moderate pain.
c. The client is in "severe" pain 3 hours after the prior medication, a narcotic, was given. Note that the order reads to give either narcotics or nonnarcotics every 3 to 4 hours. Also keep in mind that this client is within the initial 24 hours post op. Within the first 24 to 48 hours post op the client should have minimal pain so they can deep breathe and move to prevent hypostatic pneumonia. Addiction is not of concern for short periods of time. The narcotic needs to be given.
d. Nonnarcotics are for mild pain or discomforts. They are not appropriate if the client is in severe pain, especially within the initial 48 hours post op.

Test Tips

A key word in the stem is "severe" pain. Be careful not to read the "every 3 to 4 hours" time frequency for medication as "every 4 hours." If you did, you probably selected option d.

66. The correct answer is b.

Rationales

a. This is an action to take if the client has had an laminectomy.
b. These exercises will assist the venous circulation in the lower extremities. With the client in a lithotomy position, some venous stasis would have occurred.
c. This position might be used for post op venous surgery of the lower legs.
d. This position is sometimes used after arterial surgery of the legs to help promote circulation to the legs.

Test Tips

The clue in the stem is the position during the procedure—lithotomy. Think venous stasis and then read the options as you ask yourself which actions promote the venous blood to return to the heart.

67. The correct answer is c.

Rationales

a. This is an incorrect action. If done, the client will have a tendency to fall forward.

b. Elderly clients have a tendency to move into a flexion posture, so these exercises would be good for them. However, this option does not answer the question about ambulation.

c. Orthostatic reflex stimulation simply is another way of saying postural hypotension or orthostatic hypotension. Recall that as we get older the reflexes become slower. Therefore when the elderly go from a sitting to a standing position, there is a delay in the reflex of the venous system in the legs to constrict and return more blood to the heart. The client has decreased preload and, ultimately, decreased cardiac output.

d. This option is describing the effects of weight-bearing exercises in the elderly.

Test Tips

The clues in the stem are "gradual . . . ambulation." With this in mind, option c seems to be the only logical answer.

68. The correct answer is b.

Rationales

a. The verb "suppress" is a clue that this is an incorrect option. Inflammation requires elimination, not suppression.

b. Recall that an inflammation of the colon results in frequent stools from the overstimulation of peristalsis. The reduction of peri-staltic activity is the chief purpose of Banthine.

c. Use anatomy to eliminate this option. Ulcerative colitis is found mainly in the large bowel. This option focuses on the stomach, the only part of the GI tract that has mainly acidic contents.

d. Anxiety is a component of this disease in that it may trigger exacerbations. Antianxiety agents such as BuSpar might be given.

Test Tips

Banthine and Pro-Banthine are the two more common antispasmodic agents given in ulcerative colitis, bladder spasms, and gallbladder attacks. They relax the smooth muscles.

69. The correct answer is a.

Rationales

a. The lateral heel, like the lateral aspects of the fingertip, has less sensitivity than other areas. Recall that the lateral aspect of the fingertips is where blood should be obtained for glucose monitoring in clients with diabetes mellitus.

b. This is an incorrect site.

c. This is an incorrect site.

d. This is an incorrect site.

Test Tips

Associate the heel stick in a newborn with the obtaining of blood from the fingertip for glucose monitoring.

70. The correct answer is b.

Rationales

    a. This is a correct action and needs no reporting.

    b. The specifics to note in this option are that the client has an infusion pump. Actions for a gravity flow system are incorrect when applied to an infusion pump for medication administration.

    c. This is a correct action and needs no reporting.

    d. This is a correct action and needs no reporting.

Test Tips

If you read the question rapidly you may have selected a correct action instead of an incorrect action. The key words are "which action . . . is of a concern." So as you read the options, look for a wrong action.

71. The correct answer is d.

Rationales

    a. Frequent loose stools would be a later finding of amoxicillin therapy in an adult client. If the client were an infant, this would be the correct answer as the initial finding.

    b. Difficulty breathing suggests an overt finding, such as when the client is having an anaphylactic reaction.

    c. Generalized dermatitis is not an initial finding. It may occur after a rash has begun on one part of the body and then spreads.

    d. An itching rash on the abdomen is a classic initial finding for penicillin allergies of older children and adults.

Test Tips

Clues in the stem are to associate "amoxicillin" with penicillin since it is in this family of antibiotics and to note the question asks about "initial subtle manifestations." Therefore you can expect that all of the options will be untoward effects of varying degrees of severity. Use your common sense to identify an isolated area that would most likely be an initial event.

72. The correct answer is b.

Rationales

    a. This is an incomplete statement. The client also lost fluids and electrolytes through the vomiting and diarrhea.

    b. Of the given options this one is the most accurate. Be careful not to avoid this option since it includes nothing about blood. Avoid reading information into the stem. The amount of blood loss is not defined. Typically with GI distress, not hemorrhage, more fluid is lost with vomiting and diarrhea than blood.

    c. This is an incorrect statement.

    d. This is an incorrect statement. If potassium is low the bowel has a tendency to decrease peristalsis. This can be a reason for paralytic ileus.

Test Tips

Avoid focusing on the bleeding more than the vomiting and diarrhea, especially since the characteristics of the bleeding are not given. *Recall tip:* Lactated Ringer's, like 0.9% normal saline, is an isotonic fluid. It includes electrolytes and *sodium bicarbonate.* Therefore it is the fluid of choice to treat metabolic acidosis. Beware: it is usually given for 24 to 48 hours as therapy since giving it longer can result in metabolic alkalosis because of the bicarbonate.

73. The correct answer is a.

Rationales

   a. This is the correct answer. Within the first 24 to 72 hours of a burn injury there are large amounts of fluid loss and less volume in the vascular circulation. Drugs may therefore have a tendency to accumulate. After the first 72 hours the risk to the burned client is from fluid overload. Other conditions in which risk of drug accumulation occurs are left-sided congestive heart failure, shock, and pulmonary edema.
   b. This is an incorrect statement.
   c. This is an incorrect statement.
   d. This is an incorrect statement.

Test Tips

The approach to use is elimination of options that just don't sound right. For example, with option c, ask yourself: "If I had thick blood, what does that do to the Tylenol that I just took for a headache?"

74. The correct answer is d.

Rationales

   a. This antineoplastic has bone pain as an expected effect and indicates efficacy of treatment.
   b. Insomnia is not an adverse effect of this drug.
   c. Anorexia may occur as a side effect. However, it causes the client no immediate harm.
   d. Purpura of the legs is an adverse effect of this drug and indicates a possible allergic reaction. Purpura is any of several bleeding disorders characterized by hemorrhage into the tissues, particularly beneath the skin or mucous membranes, producing ecchymoses or petechiae.

Test Tips

If you have no idea of what this medication is, make an educated guess. Look at the options and put them in order of most serious to least serious. Beware: do not put bone pain as the most severe just because you have not heard much about it. When you see the word purpura think of purple skin or a bruise. This gets you thinking of bleeding, which is a priority concern with any condition. Put purpura first, then bone pain, then anorexia (since it is associated with nutrition), and insomnia last as the least important.

75. The correct answer is c.

Rationales

a. This might be the best option if the information included that the client was also on a loop diuretic, which may cause the client to lose potassium and magnesium.

b. High potassium levels have nothing to do with digitalis toxicity.

c. With hypothyroidism all medications have the risk of being metabolized slower because of the slowed metabolism. This puts the client at risk for toxicity.

d. Hyperparathyroidism results in hypercalcemia, which has no influence on toxicities.

Test Tips

Avoid reading into the question that the client is also on a potassium-losing diuretic. Note that the client is an adolescent who may not need diuretics along with the digoxin.

76. The correct answer is b.

Rationales

a. Red blood cell counts are followed when clients get Epogen, the erythropoietin recombinant. Clients with chronic renal failure in the end stage of renal failure most commonly get this drug because the kidney no longer produces erythropoietin, which stimulates the bone marrow to produce red cells.

b. Neupogen is commonly used in clients with drug-induced neutropenia. Therapeutic response is a rise in the serum blood levels of neutrophils or white blood cells and the absence of infection in the client.

c. Platelets are monitored for clients with severe infection or trauma.

d. Sedimentation rates, when elevated, indicate that an abnormal process is occurring in the body.

Test Tips

Go with what you know: associate *Neu*pogen with *neu*trophils, which are part of the white blood count. Select option b.

77. The correct answer is c.

Rationales

a. Hepatitis is either a viral or bacterial infection. It would not be the side effect of an antibiotic.

b. Arthralgia is joint pain. It is one of the side effects of beta blocker drugs.

c. Ototoxicity is the most serious side effect of streptomycin. Hearing tests need to be done when this drug is given.

d. If you read too fast you may have misread this as *nephrotoxicity* instead of *neurotoxicity*. Streptomycin does have the side effect of *nephrotoxicity* and the serum creatinine would need to be monitored.

Test Tips

Eliminate the most obvious first—hepatitis and arthralgia. Then recall that neurotoxicity is not a common side effect. Select option c.

78. The correct answer is b.

Rationales

    a. The pancreatic enzymes are monitored in severe gallbladder disease or in clients with alcoholism.

    b. Liver enzymes are logical to monitor since PO medications are metabolized through the liver.

    c. Gastric enzymes are not routinely monitored.

    d. Cardiac enzymes are monitored in clients with angina, risk of myocardial infarction, cardiac trauma, or infectious endocarditis.

Test Tips

Recall that antitubercular drug therapy usually involves the oral ingestion of two or more medications each day. Therefore it logically follows that the liver, which functions as a filtering and metabolizing plant, would be the most affected organ.

79. The correct answer is a.

Rationales

    a. Elixirs have a certain percent of alcohol in them. This is dangerous for a client on disulfiram or Antabuse. This medication and alcohol combine to cause mild to severe reactions beginning 15 minutes after the alcohol ingestion. These reactions range from flushing, headache, GI distress, sweating, and thirst to hyperventilation, respiratory difficulty, MI, CHF, convulsion, and death.

    b. Aspirin has no direct interaction with this drug.

    c. Benadryl has no direct interaction with this drug.

    d. Tylenol has no direct interaction with this drug.

Test Tips

Be careful to read the question correctly. Note that options b, c, and d should be avoided in clients with alcoholism because of their risk to damage the liver.

80. The correct answer is b.

Rationales

    a. A bright room is better for someone in delirium tremens since shadows would be minimized.

    b. A dark room leads the eyes to see more shadows. This is not good for clients that are having hallucinations, especially visual ones.

    c. Medicinal odors may be annoying to the client. They are not the most disturbing.

    d. Odors from fragrances also may be annoying to the client. However, like medicinal odors, they are not the most irritating.

Test Tips

Note the clues from the question: "which of these environmental factors" is the "most disturbing" to a client in delirium tremens. This tells you that all of the options will be environmental factors and disturbing. Your task is to put them in order of most to least and then select the most annoying factor. If you read the options to look for one correct and three incorrect options you probably had a more difficult time answering the question.

81. The correct answer is a.

Rationales

a,b,c,d. Pancreatin, a digestant, is an exogenous pancreatic enzymes replacement. It is commonly given to children with cystic fibrosis since their normal pancreatic secretions are so thick the pancreatic enzymes can't get into the GI system. The other system affected by cystic fibrosis is the pulmonary, which produces thick mucus. Therefore rigorous pulmonary toilet and the use of Mucomyst, a mucolytic to thin secretions, are essential.

Test Tips

If you automatically start to choose fats because you recall that these children have steatorrhea (fatty, foul-smelling stools), stop and think: the question is not asking that. Reword the question. The outcome increases the absorption of which substance? Of the given options, protein is the nutrient most important to the body, followed by carbohydrates, then fats, and lastly the folic and ascorbic acids. Therefore select protein.

82. The correct answer is d.

Rationales

a. Movement—or lack of it—is important when applying and removing leg braces. However, it is not the priority. Think safety to the site where the brace is used. Maintaining healthy skin without breakdown is essential to the continued use of braces on any extremity.

b. This is important but not the priority.
c. This is important but not the priority.
d. When a client has no sensation in the lower extremities, the nurse must carefully check skin integrity each time the brace is applied or removed. This skin care issue is similar for clients with diabetic neuropathy of the feet. They usually have numbness or no feeling on parts of the feet so they are taught to visually inspect their feet every day.

Test Tips

If you have no idea of the correct answer, use the cluster technique on these options. Options a, b, and c can be clustered under the umbrella of movement concerns. The odd man out, option d, concerns sensation. Select option d.

83. The correct answer is a.

Rationales

a. Forcing fluids is a priority to prevent chemical cystitis and toxicity to the kidney from the combination of drugs.

b. The antimetabolites methotrexate and fluorouracil have the side effect of photosensitivity. It is important for these clients to cover their skin with clothes. If they don't, a raised, itching rash is most likely to occur. However, hydration is a priority over protection from the sun.

c. This may be a true statement for some clients, but it is not the priority in the given situation.

d. This is an incorrect statement. The way to prevent postural hypotension, which is usually caused from an insufficient circulating volume, is to hydrate clients with fluids. The type of fluid depends upon the reason for the deficit.

Test Tips

If the presence of these three drugs confuses your thinking, simply stop and take a deep breath and take a different approach to the question and options. Think more globally. Tell yourself that when clients are on combination drug therapy (as for TB or cancer), the most important concern is to keep the drug in the circulation and get the waste products excreted. The two major excretory structures of the body are the bowel and the bladder. To keep them in good condition, fluids are essential. Select option a.

84. The correct answer is b.

Rationales

a. The need for rescue doses is not considered a complication of narcotic use for cancer pain. Rescue doses mean that in addition to the morphine drip the client might require some IV push medication to control the break through pain.

b. Small, frequent, liquid stools is a classic finding with feces impaction in the large intestine. Recall that constipation is a complication of long-term narcotic use.

c. If you read too quickly, you probably chose this as the best answer since you were thinking: narcotic and respiratory distress. Your basic thinking is correct. However, that application to this situation is incorrect. Event though the client has a respiratory rate of 10, the breathing is "deep and restful." This client has no distress. If this option stated that the breathing was "shallow and struggling" then this would be the best answer. Respiratory concerns would take priority over bowel problems.

d. A range in heart rate from 50 to 94 would be within normal parameters. A heart rate in the 50s is not uncommon during sleep.

Test Tips

The key words in the stem, "a complication of this medication regimen," guide you to focus on "complication" rather than an effect of the medication.

85. The correct answer is b.

Rationales

a. Crackles, cyanosis, and fever are suggestive of pneumonia. The fever pattern in pneumonia is usually a spike in temperature to 102 or higher.

b. Persistent fever, weight loss and night sweats are consistent with classical findings of tuberculosis (TB). The fever in TB is typically a low-grade fever of 99 or 100. Only a few other conditions have night sweats as a classic finding of the disease: Hodgkin's (lymphatic cancer, which is more common in men than in women); and acquired immunodeficiency syndrome (AIDS). Night sweats are considered as somewhat normal findings for two other situations, perimenopause and hypoglycemia during the night (an important factor for diabetics who may not have had their evening snack).

c. *Sudden* chest pain, hemoptysis (blood in the sputum), and tachycardia are classic findings in the initial stage of pulmonary embolism or infarction.

d. Nausea, diaphoresis, and severe chest pain are common findings of clients having a myocardial infarction.

Test Tips

An approach to this question is to read the options and eliminate those that you know are related to other disease conditions.

86. The correct answer is d.

Rationales

a. Eliminate this option when you acknowledge that the urine output has stabilized at about 25 ml per hour. Note the key word "sequence" before the outputs.

b. An increase in protein means the client is getting worse. However, it doesn't put the client in any immediate danger.

c. No further increase in edema is a desired effect and indicates therapy is somewhat effective.

d. The first part of the option, right-upper quadrant discomfort, is not a critical finding. However, the severe epigastric pain is a signal that the client may be in immediate danger of progressing further into eclampsia and having seizure activity. It is a classic ominous finding.

Test Tips

The clue in the stem is that it is asking for an ominous finding to be reported immediately. If you have no idea of a correct answer, use your common sense. Option d is the only option that has the word severe in it. Pay attention when you see the word severe. It is a clue to guide you to the correct answer.

87. The correct answer is a.

Rationales

a. This is the correct information for an upper GI series.

b. The option describes a version of a barium swallow where the concern is to look at the ability of the client to swallow without aspiration or regurgitation.

c. Drinking radioactive substances is not applicable to any exams of the GI tract. This is incorrect information.

d. Pictures while swallowing describes a barium swallow.

Test Tips

On questions such as these with long options, my recommendation is to closely read the options. Make your choice. Then before final selection of your answer, read the question with your selected answer one last time to validate that the information flows and fits together. Many times after reading long options you forget what the question is asking.

88. The correct answer is c.

Rationales

a. Hypercalcemia is an incorrect answer. No information given in the stem suggests a calcium problem. Hypercalcemia findings would include flaccid and weak muscle tone.

b. Hypokalemia is an incorrect answer. No information given in the stem suggests a potassium problem. Hypokalemia findings in adults would include muscle spasms, weakness, and abdominal cramps.

c. Lethargy is a finding in infants, children, and adults when the blood sugar drops suddenly and severely. Otherwise, when the glucose falls gradually the initial findings are irritability, agitation, restlessness, and hostility. If it should drop even further, confusion and lethargy occur. This is the best option since the information given in the stem was that the mother has gestational diabetes mellitus.

d. Hypoxia would be correct only if there was no information that the mother had gestational diabetes mellitus.

Test Tips

If you focused on the skin color and disregarded the level of consciousness, you probably did a knee-jerk choice of option d because it deals with oxygenation. Avoid this type of response by writing a few notes on paper to help you focus on the whole picture: lethargy, dusky, gestational diabetes, and a few hours after delivery. With these clues, think logically that the mother's insulin has crossed over into the placenta and now the neonate has insulin without a source of glucose. Recall that the neonate's liver is immature with limited glucose stores. Liver immaturity is why normal physiologic jaundice occurs 48 to 72 hours after birth.

89. The correct answer is d.

Rationales

a. This is an incorrect conclusion in the given situation. The drop in arterial oxygen pressure—what you more commonly know as the PaO_2—to a 50-mm Hg level is inappropriate for most people. At this level, most clients are considered for intubation and mechanical ventilation.

b. A physician's order is needed to change the oxygen concentration.

c. A physician's order is needed to change the oxygen concentration and repeat lab tests.

d. Of the given options, this one—to check the client and communicate the overall condition of the client to the physician—is the best since it is the most comprehensive.

Test Tips

Apply the nursing process to select the best answer. Think like this: the client's therapy changed, changes occurred in the labs, so do further assessment rather than an intervention. Options that describe further assessment are commonly the best answers when client problems occur. If the question included information indicating that the client was in respiratory distress or arrest, then the correct answer would be b.

90. The correct answer is d.

Rationales
   a. This option would be correct if the information was given that the client had a drinking binge 48 to 72 hours prior to hospitalization.
   b. This option would be correct if the client was not started on a tranquilizer.
   c. Thiamine has nothing to do with controlling or preventing delirium tremens (DTs). Thiamine is given to enhance overall body and liver function.
   d. The risk is minimal for DTs since the client was started on tranquilizers.

Test Tips

Avoid knee-jerk reactions based on information that you know. If you chose option b upon initially reading the options, the best suggestion is for you to read the options in reverse: jump to option d and read it, followed by option c. Read the options in reverse order so you pay full attention to what is presented. Otherwise, if you know option b is the answer and

then read in a sequence of option c then d, you tend to gloss over the remaining options. Another suggestion for when much information is given in the stem (as in this question) is to jot down a few notes as if taking a report.

91. The correct answer is d.

Rationales
   a. This is an incorrect angle.
   b. This is an incorrect angle.
   c. This is an incorrect angle.
   d. This is a correct angle to insert the needle into an implanted venous access device or implanted-infusion port.

Test Tips

If you are unfamiliar with this device, the recommendation is to look up a picture of it in your textbook. The visual stimulation will help you better remember the specifics of care with this device. If you have no idea of the correct answer, use common sense. Think of a device under the skin. To best stick a needle into it and be sure you are at the site, palpate the device and use a 90-degree angle. The same technique is used for arterial sticks that are done by palpation.

92. The correct answer is b.

Rationales
   a. This intervention would be the third item of importance.
   b. This is the priority since the central total parenteral nutrition is a high glucose solution of usually about 25% and the client was just started on the solution. If the in-

formation in the stem was different (for example, to focus on the nutritional status of the client), then daily weights would be the correct answer.

   c. Daily weights are the last item on the list of priorities for this question. Weights are taken to identify if the solution is meeting the client's nutritional needs. No more than a gain of 2 pounds a week is usually recommended.

   d. This is the second item in the list of priorities for this given situation.

Test Tips
The fact that the therapy has started is important to guide how you prioritize the options. When the question asks the "highest priority," assume that all of the options will be correct. If you looked for incorrect options you were using an incorrect approach to this question.

93. The correct answer is a.

Rationales
   a. Pneumonia is an infection. Erythromycin is the best answer since it is the only antibiotic listed.

   b. Adrenalin, a bronchodilator, might be the answer if the information included that the client had severe respiratory distress.

   c. Rifampin, an antitubercular agent, has nothing to do with pneumonia.

   d. Aminophylline, a theophylline bronchodilator, would be used if the client had a history of asthma and respiratory distress.

Test Tips
The clue in the stem is pneumonia, which is typically caused by a bacteria or a virus. In either case the most prescribed agent would be an antibiotic. The key to the correct answer is to put each of the drugs in their drug classification. Select option a. Avoid the process of selecting option a and then not reading the other options. If you have this habit, force yourself to change your sequence of option reading. Read option a, then d, c, and b. You will give closer attention to the information given in each option.

94. The correct answer is c.

Rationales
   a. Care for teeth is done with sterile technique or surgical asepsis. There is no concern for a dirty environment or equipment.

   b. The situation of a hematoma is one where the skin is unbroken and therefore the risk of tetanus in minimal.

   c. A cut results in deeper tissue damage. The broken bottle on the beach is similar to a rusty nail—it has the potential to cause tetanus since it is likely to be dirty.

   d. A scratch is superficial tissue damage. Even though the wood fence may cause a threat of tetanus it is unlikely since the trauma in this case is superficial.

Test Tips
If you narrowed the options to c and d, you are doing well. Now use your com-

mon sense that a cut is deeper than a scratch. Select the situation with a cut. Both objects are considered dirty, so base your decision on the depth and severity of the skin damage rather than on the object that caused it.

95. The correct answer is d.

Rationales
a. Control of fat intake is most important with gallbladder problems.
b. Vegetarians would restrict their intake of animal fats.
c. Increased calories are critical for clients who have anorexia nervosa, who are getting chemotherapy for cancer, or who have burns.
d. Concentrated carbohydrates (CHO) pull water into the intestinal tract, distend it, and then produce cramping and watery stools. This dumping syndrome is the result of partial gastrectomies—Billroth I or II. The food is dumped into the small intestine quickly since the stomach is smaller. Then the process described above occurs.

Test Tips
Associate that too much CHO for clients with COPD will result in acute respiratory distress findings. When CHO are broken down they give off large amounts of CO_2 as a byproduct. Obviously, the higher levels of CO_2 increase the workload for clients with COPD. Within 2 to 3 hours after eating a meal that is rich in CHO they may have acute respiratory distress.

96. The correct answer is c.

Rationales
a. This information is irrelevant to the given situation.
b. This information is irrelevant to the given situation.
c. Belladonna, an anticholinergic, is used to prevent or treat bladder spasms that occur after bladder surgery. It also has the action of dilating the pupils, just like atropine. Pupil dilation is to be aoided if glaucoma is present. Dilation of the pupil can cause acute glaucoma manifested by acute eye pain.
d. This information is irrelevant to the given situation.

Test Tips
If you have no idea of the correct answer, use the option cluster technique. Group options a, b, and d under a history of these conditions. The odd man out, c, deals with current medications and the current time. Select it.

97. The correct answer is b.

Rationales
a. This is an incorrect action.
b. The client is toxic, based on this blood level. Anything over 20 is considered a toxic level. The client may have findings of nausea, muscle twitching, and a heart rate over 120. As a rule of thumb, however, use client complaints or symptoms as a measure of toxicity, not just lab values.

c. IV rates are not routinely changed without a physician order. Be aware that some agencies have a standard that IV fluids without medications can be adjusted by 10 percent until the physician is notified. However, this rule is not generally accepted nationally.

d. No information is given to support the need to repeat the blood level. If there was difficulty getting the blood and it hemolyzed, then a repeat test is appropriate.

Test Tips

If you are not sure of the answer, and narrowed the options to a or b, go with the safest approach. Notify the physician.

98. The correct answer is c.

Rationales

a. An increase in a heart rate by 10 would not be significant in the given situation of shock.

b. The words "sustained decrease" indicate that the output has stabilized at 25 ml per hour and there is no further drop.

c. A blood pressure for any client should be maintained minimally at 90 systolic. This drop is significant since the situation is that the client is already in shock—the decompensation stage.

d. A change in respiratory rate is more important in pulmonary conditions than in cardiovascular conditions.

Test Tips

If you missed the fact that the client is already in shock, you were probably looking for initial findings of shock so you chose option a. Note that the question is asking for findings of "progressing further" in the shock state.

99. The correct answer is a.

Rationales

a. Anergy is an immunodeficient condition characterized by a lack of or diminished reaction to an antigen or group of antigens. This state may be seen in advanced TB, AIDS, and in some malignancies.

b. This would be a positive finding in 48 to 72 hours for a person with no immune problems.

c. This would be a negative finding in 48 to 72 hours for a person with no immune problems.

d. This would be a positive finding in 48 to 72 hours for a person with no immune problems.

Test Tips

An induration is a hardened, raised, red area measured by diameter. If you had no idea of a correct answer, you could use the option cluster technique. Cluster options b, c, and d, since they have numbers associated with them. Choose the odd man out; the option without numbers.

100. The correct answer is c.

Rationales

a. This is an appropriate action. However, it is not the priority action.

b. Dangling on the side of the bed is one position for a paracentesis. However, it is neither the only position nor the priority for instruction.
c. An empty bladder is essential for the prevention of a bladder puncture during the procedure. This instruction is the priority.
d. This is an appropriate position for this procedure. It is not the priority for instruction.

Test Tips

When answering a question such as this (where all of the options are correct instructions), for each option ask yourself: What is the worst thing that can happen if I don't do this? The worst outcome is in option c, a punctured bladder. Therefore it is most likely the priority.

101. The correct answer is a.

Rationales

a. Low potassium results in leg cramps, abdominal cramps, and feelings of weakness.
b. Magnesium may also cause leg cramps but this is not as likely to result from the loop diuretics.
c. Calcium loss is not a factor associated with diuretic use.
d. Protein loss is not a factor associated with diuretic use.

Test Tips

If you are not sure of the correct answer, go with what you know. Potassium changes are more commonly associated with the effect of diuretics.

102. The correct answer is c.

Rationales

a. A change in stool consistency may indicate effectiveness of antibiotics, which are given for some types of bowel infections. However, it is not the best answer since it would be a day or two before the client might have a bowel movement.
b. Antibiotics don't relieve pain directly. Indirectly they might reduce inflammation, which then reduces the pain.
c. A temperature drop of 2 degrees is an objective and faster way to determine if an antibiotic is effective.
d. Even though urine is clear, a pungent odor would cause concern and a need for further monitoring.

Test Tips

If you have no idea of a correct answer, go with what you know. Think of the situation of infection. The most common objective parameter used to determine infection is a rise in temperature. It logically follows that a way to tell if infection is on the wane is to monitor temperature for a drop.

103. The correct answer is c.

Rationales

a. This is a false statement. Clients with asthma need to force fluids to liquefy pulmonary secretions.
b. This is a false statement. There are other factors that can stimulate an asthma attack.

c. The sputum of clients with asthma is thicker than normal. They also have narrowed airways due to bronchial constriction.

d. The time frame makes this an incorrect statement. Not all clients with asthma improve *quickly*.

Test Tips

Careful reading will help you avoid an incorrect answer. Option b sounds correct. Beware: this is an example of an absolute statement. You have heard about absolute words (for example, never, always, and every) and now you have been introduced to an absolute statement. As written this means that nothing else other than anxiety causes asthma attacks. This is a false statement.

104. The correct answer is d.

Rationales

a. Prone position is lying face down. It is an incorrect position for a client in respiratory distress.

b. Supine position is lying flat with the face up. This is a position for some x-ray procedures, a resting ECG, and an EEG.

c. Trendelenburg is the position for a pregnant client whose cord has prolapsed after her water has broken. Modified Trendelenburg (head flat and legs elevated at least 45 degrees) is the position for a client in shock.

d. The client's preferred position is the best position for this client.

Test Tips

If you have no idea of a correct answer, simply select the option that is client centered, option d.

105. The correct answer is c.

Rationales

a. Respiratory rate is a priority if no other variable is given for evaluation of progress in a respiratory condition.

b. Breath sounds give information as to the degree of bronchial and alveolar opening or collapse. It would be third in priority for the evaluation of a client's overall condition.

c. Respiratory effort is the priority for an overall evaluation of progress of therapy for clients with asthma.

d. The normal inspiratory/expiratory ratio is 1:2. In clients with COPD it is greater (for example, 1:3 or 1:4).

Test Tips

Remember that with increased respiratory effort the client can maintain normal parameters such as respiratory rate, depth, and rhythm.

106. The correct answer is a.

Rationales

a. The use of a pain scale is the most objective way to evaluate the severity of a client's pain. It can be used even if the prior nurse did not use it. Define the scale to the client—numbers 1 to 10, with 10 being the most severe pain and 1 being the least. Ask the client where the current pain falls on the scale. Then ask where the pain experienced with the prior medication fell. This same process can be used with clients who have respiratory distress.

b. There is no such thing as a subjective pain scale.

c. Asking if it is more or less is an appropriate approach, but not the best approach. This question can be put under the pain scale method. Once the client identifies a number, ask if the pain is more or less than the prior number.

d. Checking to see how much pain medication the client has received is an appropriate action. However, it does not best answer the question.

Test Tips

When one option can be an umbrella for one or more of the other options it is usually the best answer. Option a can be an umbrella for option c. Refer to the discussion in Rationales. Therefore option a is the best answer.

107. The correct answer is a.

Rationales

a. When clients with renal problems are encouraged to force fluids, clear liquids are the fluid of choice. Water is the best choice of the given options since the client is on a sulfonamide. Sulfonamides are more effective in alkaline urine than in acidic urine. Therefore acidic fluids should be avoided if the sulfonamide is given for urinary infections. If sulfonamides are given for ear infection or bowel inflammation, the type of fluid is of no concern.

b. Apple juice may make the urine more acidic and the sulfonamide less effective. Therefore it is not the best choice.

c. Orange juice may make the urine more acidic and the sulfonamide less effective. Therefore it is not the best choice.

d. Hot chocolate is not a good choice since it has cocoa and may further irritate the urinary system.

Test Tips

If you had trouble deciding between orange and apple juice, remember this clue: if two options are very similar, then the correct answer is probably another option. Reread the information and the options. The sulfonamides are unique in that they are more effective in urine with a higher pH.

108. The correct answer is c.

Rationales

a. Goggles will only protect the eyes. The face also needs protection from the potential secretions from the new trach—especially when the client coughs. Coughing with a tracheostomy opening allows for the sputum to be spewed forcefully in every direction.

b. With only gown and gloves there is no face protection. Remember that the nurse will be leaning over the client to perform the dressing change and trach care.

c. This is the best approach to protecting both the nurse and the client from infection.

d. Gloves are absent from this option, which makes it incorrect.

Test Tips

Both the nurse and the client must be protected during dressing changes. A new trach may have fresh oozing of serosanguineous drainage and increased secretions from the stimulation of the respiratory tract by the trach tube, which acts as a foreign object. Minimally, gloves and a mask with a face shield need to be worn.

109. The correct answer is d.

Rationales

a. Being hungry and having peristalsis of the bowel can be separate occurrences. This is not the best answer.

b. Ambulation helps to promote peristalsis. Be careful not to think that when you ambulate you have peristalsis. This is a false assumption.

c. In many institutions the rule is that when the IV comes out, the client can eat. This is not physiologically correct. Avoid selection of answers based on an agency's protocol. Usually it is an incorrect answer.

d. When the client can tolerate clear liquids it is an indication that the bowel has sufficient peristalsis for heavier, more complex foods.

Test Tips

If you have no idea of the correct answer, go with what you know and have learned in basic post operative care. If the client tolerates one type of diet, advance them to the next level of foodstuffs.

110. The correct answer is d.

Rationales

a. Leukemia has no association with levels of low potassium.

b. Bacteria in the urine is not a standard finding of persons with leukemia. Note that this option introduces new information of an infection. When options introduce new information not mentioned in the stem they are often not the correct answers (as is in this case).

c. High glucose may be found in clients with high stress since the sympathetic system stimulates the breakdown of the glycogen stores in the liver to glucose. No information is given that this client is under high stress. Also glucose has no direct association with the condition of leukemia.

d. A low platelet count is a common finding of clients with leukemia. Thus they may have bleeding problems and easy bruising.

Test Tips

If you are not sure of the correct answer, think first of the pathophysiology of leukemia. Leukemia is a proliferation of immature white cells, which are over-produced in the bone marrow. Next think of what other cells are producing in the bone marrow. They are the red cells and the platelets. Of the given options, the only one listed is the platelets. Select it. Both of these levels are typically low since the bone marrow is exhausted from producing the immature white cells and little ability is left to produce red cells and platelets.

111. The correct answer is d.

Rationales

    a. Needing to be like your peers is most characteristic of the teen years.

    b. The key word that makes this option incorrect is "peak." Separation anxiety is still present at age 6 but it is not at its peak, as it is in the toddler (1 to 3 years of age).

    c. An increased need for privacy is seen in the teen years.

    d. This is the answer that best describes the developmental characteristics of a 6-year-old who is at the end of being a preschooler and on the cusp of being a school-age child.

Test Tips

The most common error on this question is to misread option b. The key phrase "at its peak" may be read but not really acknowledged. The two options that are chosen with difficulty are options b and d. If this happened to you, use the techniques to read the second part of the statement first. For example, the peak of separation anxiety is at this time. Then you will be able to find your error in reading and selection of the correct option will be made easier.

112. The correct answer is d.

Rationales

    a. An MRI, a noninvasive procedure, is done to find tumors, foreign objects, cancers, or other abnormalities of organs or the bones. It becomes invasive if it is ordered with a contrast.

    b. A chest x-ray, a noninvasive procedure, provides for the location of tumors and determination of heart failure and infectious processes such as pneumonia.

    c. A lumbar puncture, an invasive procedure, allows for decisions regarding the type of medication used to treat infections such as meningitis.

    d. Bone marrow aspiration, an invasive procedure, assists with the diagnosis of leukemia and bone cancer.

Test Tips

If you have no idea of the correct answer, associate leukemia with the white blood cells that are produced in the bone marrow. Match your thoughts with the option d.

113. The correct answer is b.

Rationales
   a. Urine output is associated with cardiovascular status, not infectious processes.
   b. A normal body temperature indicates the freedom from infection.
   c. Frequency of the visits from the parents has no relationship to infections or freedom from infection.
   d. This option sounds good since most people as they read it think of a decrease in the white blood count. However, read a little closer. The key word "change" gives no direction of the change. Thus this option is too general and is incorrect. The word "change" is a red flag word like the word "severe." Pay closer attention when you find these words in the stem or the options.

Test Tips
Key words in the stem are "remain free from infection." This guides you to select a normal finding.

114. The correct answer is c.

Rationales
   a. This rate is too slow for a fetus.
   b. This rate is also too slow for a fetus.
   c. This is the correct answer. A fetal heart rate is similar to that of the infant—120 to 160 beats per minute at any time in the pregnancy.
   d. This rate is too fast for a fetus.

Test Tips
For this question try the "eliminate extremes" approach. Eliminate options a and d since they are the extremes. Since the question is about a fetus select the higher rate of 140. If the question was about an adult with a problem or the pregnant mother, then I would select lower rate of 110 beats per minute.

115. The correct answer is c.

Rationales
   a. This option does not answer the question about the goal of the "baby's care."
   b. This option does not answer the question about the goal of the "baby's care."
   c. This option directly addresses the goal for the "baby's care."
   d. This option does not answer the question about the goal of the "baby's care." If the question asked about the long-term goal without being specific, then this option would be the best of the given options.

Test Tips
If you are trying to decide between any two of these options, go back to the question, which usually holds the clues to option selection. Avoid focusing on long-term goals. Rather, focus on how they define the goal—it's about the baby. Then reread the options and select the one about the baby.

116. The correct answer is a.

Rationales

a. This is the correct option. A pregnant woman needs at least 1½ times as much calcium as a nonpregnant woman.

b. Pregnant women are not to drink any alcoholic beverages. Alcohol can cause fetal abnormalities when as little as 8 ounces of beer a day is consumed.

c. Decreasing fluid intake in the evening is recommended only if the mother has the problem of frequent urination at night associated with drinking fluids in the evening.

d. On first reading, this option sounds correct. However, it is an incorrect statement. It is the craving of nonfood substances, not food, which indicates a nutritional abnormality. These cravings are called pica and indicate a deficiency in the woman's iron, of which she needs twice the normal daily amount during pregnancy. Food cravings are a normal phenomenon in pregnancy.

Test Tips

If you narrowed the options to a and d, reread the question. The focus is on helping the client choose proper foods. Therefore option a is more in line with the question than option d, which is focused on nutritional deficiencies.

117. The correct answer is c.

Rationales

a. This is a false statement.

b. The client will not be alone. However, the client will be doing the work of labor.

c. Breathing techniques are practiced long before the actual delivery process. Two types of breathing practiced are deep, slow, rhythmic breathing; and panting, which is short, shallow, and rhythmic.

d. This option has the absolute word "all" in it, so put your antennas up. It makes this option incorrect.

Test Tips

If you have no idea of the correct answer, you can cluster the options under the umbrella of self-centeredness. Options a, b, and d focus on the "I," whereas option c is a logical statement. Select option c.

118. The correct answer is d.

Rationales

a. This statement does not indicate potential danger. Note in the stem that the stabbing is associated with the neighbor.

b. It is of a concern what the voices are telling the client. However, related to this particular statement, it is of a lesser concern for the nurse, since the client is a danger only to himself.

c. This statement is one where the client changed the subject. Of course the client, being actively psychotic, would most likely not be allowed to shower. Shaving with a battery razor may be allowed; a safety razor or razor with electric cord may be avoided for fear the client would harm himself.

d. This statement is of most concern since not only is the client in danger but others around the client may also be threatened if the voices tell him to harm others.

Test Tips
Compare the verbs in the options: "I want," "are telling," "I want," and "I will." Just from looking at these you can identify that the strongest statement is the last option. Sometimes if you cannot find any other clue compare the verbs in the options then reread the question to clarify what is being asked.

119. The correct answer is b.

Rationales

a. This would be a correct option if the time frame was "on admission to the unit."

b. This is the best approach since the question is asking about "as his condition improves."

c. This approach is incorrect and would be used only if information was given in the stem that the client had a cognitive impairment of some type.

d. This approach would be used prior to discharge or after discharge. It allows more freedom and at that point the client would hopefully be able to handle it.

Test Tips
If you focused on the diagnosis you most likely missed valuable information about the progress of the client ("as his condition improves"). On any question keep in mind the time frame. Remember, you only see what you look for. Be on alert for time frames; they offer valuable clues.

120. The correct answer is d.

Rationales

a. Negating a client's hallucination is an inappropriate action.

b. Asking the client to prove voices are real is also an incorrect action.

c. Group activity is inappropriate for clients who exhibit behaviors that are out of touch with reality. A psychotic client needs to be separated from others and observed closely by the staff.

d. When a client has erratic behavior, no matter what the cause, an appropriate approach is to comment or focus on the emotions tied to the behavior. The behavior is played down.

Test Tips
Be careful to read the stem correctly for "auditory" hallucinations. If you had no idea of a correct answer, go with the option that is a most realistic action to deal

with the voices. This approach eliminates option c immediately, since it ignores the voices. Of the remaining options the most realistic one is option d.

121. The correct answer is b.

Rationales
    a. Nausea is a good choice if the question asks about a medication in general, since it is usually a first sign of drug intolerance.
    b. Apply what you know about most of the psychotropic drugs; drowsiness is a side effect.
    c. Avoid misreading this option as hypotension instead of hypertension. Hypotension, like drowsiness, is a common side effect of psychotropic drugs. The specific type is postural hypotension.
    d. Frequent urination is a finding associated with a urinary tract infection, hyperglycemia, diabetes mellitus, or ketoacidosis and of a distended bladder.

Test Tips
You can think this question through to get the correct answer if you had trouble with your recall. Note that an antipsychotic drug is given to psychotic persons to bring them back to reality. Often these clients are hyperactive in some manner, either physically or verbally. So an intent of the medication is to slow them down. The only option that might be associated with a slowing down is option b, drowsiness.

122. The correct answer is a.

Rationales
    a. These characteristics are classic findings for pulmonary edema.
    b. Clear, white, or thin sputum are normal features. Note that white secretions from the eyes or nose might indicate allergies.
    c. Brown or gray-colored sputum suggests the presence of old blood or a history of smoke inhalation.
    d. Yellow or green and thick sputum are typically found with bacterial pneumonia.

Test Tips
The clue is in the question—pulmonary edema. Note that if the given condition is changed, then the correct answer also changes.

123. The correct answer is a.

Rationales
    a. Bran cereal will prevent constipation, a common complication of long-term narcotic use.
    b. Rice has a potential constipating effect with some people. Thus it is not the best answer.
    c. Peanut butter commonly puts persons at risk for constipation.
    d. Cheese enhances the possibility of constipation.

Test Tips
If you have no idea of the correct answer, attempt to reword the question. As stated, this question is convoluted and confusing.

A rewording might be, which of these foods will not cause respiratory distress, constipation, or urine retention? Note that I substituted the actual complications of narcotic analgesics. As you read the options you realize that the only one of these focused on is constipation. Go with what you know, that bran stimulates the bowel to promote peristalsis and regular bowel movements.

124. The correct answer is c.

Rationales

 a. This option introduces new information into the situation. It is not the correct answer.
 b. The first part of this option might be an approach to handling the situation—wait 5 minutes for the client to get less anxious. However, the reason for the anxiety is new information not given in the stem. Therefore the new information makes it an incorrect option.
 c. Notification of the physician is the right action to take at this time.
 d. This is incorrect. The physician is the one to order the rescheduling if the procedure is thought to be essential to the care of the client. Sometimes clients will reschedule the date of procedures. However, there is not enough information in the stem to select this as a correct option.

Test Tips
Avoid the selection of options that introduce new information into the situation when the other options don't. Also remember your common sense and logical thinking. When there is a client problem, stabilize the client and notify the physician.

125. The correct answer is c.

Rationales

 a. A client with obsessive-compulsive behavior may not have a behavior that is disturbing to another, so a semiprivate room would be satisfactory.
 b. A depressed client moves and talks very little, so a semiprivate room is appropriate.
 c. Usually clients with a bipolar diagnosis are admitted in the manic state. Recall that they move a lot and talk a lot. These behaviors would be most disturbing to another client. A last factor to consider is that these clients may be out of touch with reality and have the potential to harm others.
 d. Clients with borderline personality would be a second choice for a private room. Recall that usual characteristics are splitting (seeing things as all good or all bad), increased risk of danger to self, poor judgment, impulsivity with inappropriate and intense anger, and extreme and rapid mood changes.

Test Tips
If you narrowed the options to c and d you are on the right track. Option c is the best answer, since the bipolar client

in a manic state is at higher risk to harm others than the client with borderline personality.

126. The correct answer is b.

Rationales

a. This client is independent per activities and doesn't need the call light within reach. If you selected this option you made a knee-jerk choice rather than thinking about the given information in the stem. I recommend that next time you write down a few notes as if you were taking a nursing report.

b. Having the bed in low position is the best answer. Think logically, and think of yourself getting out of bed at night. First you get out of bed, then you walk to the bathroom. Therefore the bed being low is more important than a light being on.

c. Turning the light on would be a good second action.

d. Extension of the oxygen tube would pose a threat to safety. Besides a client that is on 3 liters/min probably can tolerate being off of the oxygen while in the bathroom.

Test Tips

To make your decision easier on these types of questions, ask yourself what is the worst thing that would happen if the action was not done? In option a (without a call light), the nurse would not be notified when the client got out of bed. No matter, since the client is independent. In option b (bed not in the low position), the client would most likely fall out of the bed. In option c (night light not on) the client would probably bump into the furniture and get a little bruised. In option d (client not have oxygen tubing), the client would probably do fine since it is at such a low dose. With this approach it is evident that option b is the best in the given situation.

127. The correct answer is d.

Rationales

a. The daytime routine is not of a priority since the daytime routine will be disrupted by lab testing, procedures, different meal times, etc.

b. Toilet training is not of primary importance since most people and children admitted to a hospital regress. Even if the child was potty trained at home the toddler will most likely revert to the diaper stage in the hospital.

c. Communication style initially sounds great until you read the second part first—the child's style of communication. This mean more than just what words the child uses or says for what items. Style includes nonverbal movements and verbal words, pitch, tone, and the emotion behind statements. Thus it is too global an option to be the best answer.

d. Bedtime routine is the priority information to obtain. By evening most of the day's activity will wane. Rituals for bedtime may be carried out without interruption.

Test Tips
If you missed this question, it probably was from the error of not reading and acknowledging the second word in each option. To prevent this error simply read each option with two words backwards.

128. The correct answer is b.

Rationales
a. Soap is helpful but is not the most important item.
b. Friction is the most important item in a handwashing routine.
c. Paper towels are not the most important item.
d. The temperature of the water is not critical. The temperature is more of a comfort for the person washing his or her hands.

Test Tips
This is a classic easy question. Make a note of it and don't miss the easy ones.

129. The correct answer is a.

Rationales
a. First identify that the medication to be started is a catecholamine which basically has actions similar to epinephrine. The initial action, therefore, will be to check the cardiovascular system. After the medication is started for 15 minutes it is reasonable to recheck the parameters that you got as a baseline. Dopamine is used to treat chronic heart failure.

b. The respiratory system is not the target organ of this medication. This is an incorrect parameter to check.
c. This option reads as if the physician had given further orders. Do not select it since it introduces new information into the situation. The actions themselves are appropriate but only with orders.
d. The only difference between this option and option a are a few key words. It is incorrect to check the "earlier" blood pressure and heart rate. A current parameter is needed. A second item that makes this option incorrect is the recheck in "1 hour." This is much too long a wait to evaluate the effectiveness or complications of the drug.

Test Tips
The best approach to help keep the information clear in your mind for the options is to read vertically for each set of items. For example, start out with check BP and HR, check respiratory, check vital signs, check "prior" BP and HR. At this point eliminate options b and d since they are not appropriate for first actions. Remember that the question is not only asking for actions but also for the sequence of actions.

130. The correct answer is b.

Rationales
a. This is an incorrect answer.
b. This is the correct answer since in leukemia white cells proliferate

and they are immature. Thus the body is unable to be protected from infections.

c. This is an incorrect answer.

d. This is an incorrect answer. The platelets are low, not high, in leukemia.

Test Tips

Do you think that you have seen this question before? Yes, you have seen this exact question earlier in this test. However, the options have been changed. If you read too quickly the tendency is to select platelets without seeing that there is a "high" before it. Read carefully. Many exams will have similar questions with similar stems or options.

131. The correct answer is d.

Rationales

a. The flank is the site of a renal biopsy.

b. The right upper quadrant could be the site of a liver biopsy.

c. The lower lumbar area is not a site for any particular test.

d. The iliac crest is the common site for a bone marrow aspiration. Other sites include the sternum and the posterior pelvic bone.

Test Tips

Associate anatomy with each site to help with your decision-making. Think: Flank is kidney; right upper quadrant is liver or gallbladder; the lower lumbar area is where low back pain commonly occurs

from back strain from heavy lifting, pregnancy or middle-age spread; iliac crest is bone, a typical place to obtain bone marrow.

132. The correct answer is b.

Rationales

a. This is a low hemoglobin but not one of great concern. A hemoglobin of 8 or lower is one that needs to be reported to the physician.

b. This elevated PTT is of concern since it is 1½ times that of the normal 30. Recall that the liver is one of the more vascular organs. The information in the stem states that a biopsy is scheduled in 2 days. With the PTT elevated the client is at risk for hemorrhage during or after the procedure.

c. An elevated blood urea nitrogen (BUN) indicates an increased breakdown of protein in the body. Reasons could be that the client has blood in the gastrointestinal tract, has eaten a meal high in protein, is dehydrated, or is breaking down the client's own muscle mass.

d. An elevated ammonia level indicates that the liver is in some degree of failure. It is unable to convert ammonia, a by-product of protein breakdown, into urea to be excreted through the kidneys. Without further information this finding means little.

Test Tips

When you narrow the options to either a or b, think pathophysiologically. A low hemoglobin means anemia, a chronic condition. An elevated PTT means a threat of bleeding and hemorrhage, an acute condition. Select option b, which puts the client in more immediate danger, especially with an invasive test being scheduled in two days.

133. The correct answer is b.

Rationales

    a. This client requires close attention to the arterial site and for the staff member to have knowledge of the complications and required actions since it involves an artery.

    b. A tomogram is similar to an x-ray except that it can distinguish between a fluid and a tissue-filled space. It is not invasive. It is the most appropriate to assign to a nursing tech.

    c. This client requires the skill of a licensed person, either RN or LVN, since the risk of eclampsia exists.

    d. This client most likely is nervous and will have many questions. A licensed person would best be able to give the required support and education.

Test Tips

If you are confused about the selection of the best answer, use the cluster technique with the umbrella of "what clients will need education?" The one that doesn't is the one most likely to be assigned to the nursing assistant.

134. The correct answer is c.

Rationales

    a. This is an incorrect answer.

    b. Wetting of the bed (enuresis) is why tricyclics are given to children.

    c. As with many medications, the effect on children is the opposite of what happens to adults. This is the correct answer.

    d. This is an incorrect answer.

Test Tips

Avoid getting stuck on the fact that a child is on an antidepressant. Look beyond that to the actual question of what might be the side effect. Go with what you know: Think of drugs for attention deficit disorders in children. In adults these drugs have a stimulation effect; in children they have a calming effect.

135. The correct answer is a.

Rationales

    a. Persistent constipation indicates that the amount of the Synthroid is deficient since the client has a finding of hypothyroidism.

    b. This sounds good as an option. Note the word "changes." The option does not give information as to the types or direction of the changes. Has sleep improved or gotten worse?

    c. This action is for clients who have permanent pacemakers. Their pulse should be at least the rate that the pacemaker is set at (usually 50 to 60 beats per minute).

d. This sounds good as an option. Note the word "changes." The option does not give information as to the types or direction of the changes. Have energy levels improved or gotten worse?

Test Tips

Identify the correct answer by rereading the options to eliminate those that are wrong. Avoid selection of options with the word "change" in them unless the direction of the change is specified.

136. The correct answer is d.

Rationales
a. This is not associated with accidents in the elderly.
b. This is not associated with accidents in the elderly.
c. This is not associated with accidents in the elderly.
d. Decreased sensory acuity in the elderly includes the senses of hearing, sight, and touch. Even thought the factors in options a, b, and c may indirectly impact the risk of accidents in the elderly, they are not a direct impact as are sensory decreases.

Test Tips

Eliminate options a and b, since they are specific to the brain's functioning. Note that the question is more of a general than a specific question. Of the remaining options c and d, select option d since it has the direction of the alteration. Note that option c simply states "altered nutritional status." It gives no direction if it is a decreased or increased problem.

137. The correct answer is d.

Rationales
a. Apples contain no high levels of electrolytes, which are harmful in clients with renal failure.
b. Dried fruits contain no high levels of electrolytes, which are harmful in clients with renal failure.
c. Cranberries contain no high levels of electrolytes, which are harmful in clients with renal failure.
d. Apricots contain high levels of potassium.

Test Tips

A difficulty with this question is the wording. A few test questions on any test are similar to this type of question. Reword the question: What food is to be taken minimally?

138. The correct answer is b.

Rationales
a. As long as a client is verbal and can be heard, the staff knows that the client is minimally functioning.
b. An IV is a priority to check since it is going into the body internally. If you avoided selecting this option since in your experience the beeping IVs are checked later, keep in mind the situation given in this question. You have no idea of what the fluid is or if the site is peripheral or central.

c. If you thought hemorrhage when you read this option, you are on the right track. Now think of characteristics of the client in shock. Now reread the option. Note that clients in shock do not typically put their light on to tell of drainage increases. This is called the use of common sense.

d. Note the tense and the time of the reported reaction. Therefore it is not a priority now.

Test Tips

This question is at the higher level of testing, the application questions. The main focus for you is to not get disturbed or upset with these types of questions. Control your emotional response by deep breathing, imagery, mini-vacations, or by simply leaving the room for a few minutes. And when you do, remember to move your muscles to indirectly stimulate your mind.

139. The correct answer is d.

Rationales

a. Avoid being fooled by the chicken. Broth is just that; is contains no meat of the chicken.

b. Potatoes provide carbohydrates and electrolytes.

c. Avocados are high in fat and vitamin B_6.

d. Tapioca pudding has protein from the milk used in the pudding.

Test Tips

Avoid reading into the options. Use some common sense. Reread the question to refocus yourself on what is being asked.

140. The correct answer is b.

Rationales

a. An incorrect sequence is not detrimental to the client.

b. Atropine for tachycardia is detrimental to the client since atropine has the effect of increasing the rate and the conduction of the impulse through the heart. This action may cause the client to have a cardiac arrest from overstimulation.

c. A too-short needle for an IM injection is not harmful to the client.

d. This mixes the insulin in the bottle in a different manner. It would not be harmful to the client.

Test Tip

Use the approach with each option to ask what is the worst thing that could happen if the nurse had that action. The action most harmful to the client is the correct answer.

141. The correct answer is a.

Rationales

a. Another client with leukemia is the best choice of the given options. Remember the ABCS—safety is the priority concern since the child falls into category of being immunosuppressed. With leu-

kemia the large volume of immature white cells does not provide protection from infection. The age would be the second item to match if it were possible. In this case it is not possible to match the client to the same age group because of the risk of infection.
b. This child with tuberculosis is an infectious threat to the client's safety.
c. Intestinal inflammation is a potential source of infection to the child with leukemia.
d. Influenza is a highly contagious infection of the respiratory tract caused by a myxovirus and other strains of virus and transmitted by airborne droplet infection. This roommate is inappropriate for a client considered immunosuppressed.

Test Tips

With immunosuppressed clients selecting a roommate without an infectious process is the priority over matching the age group. In this case group the options b, c, and d as clients with infection.

142. The correct answer is c.

Rationales

a. If a client is screaming of pain, the assumption is that the vital signs are minimally acceptable.
b. A client with an IV beeping has no indication for checking the vital signs.
c. The client that has increased drainage on a dressing may be at risk for the development of shock.

It is a priority to check the vital signs, compare them to the prior set, and look for a sustained increased heart rate of 20 over the prior rate. This would be an initial indication of shock.
d. If the client had a reaction on the last shift, it would not be a priority to get the vital signs before the client in option c.

Test Tips

Think of the need for vital signs in situations of potential shock, allergic reactions, and severe changes in a client's status. Of the given options the client with the potential for shock takes precedence.

143. The correct answer is b.

Rationales

a. Since the stem gives no information about the skill level of the patient care assistant (PCA), assignment to a dressing change is incorrect. If the stem included that the PCA was a graduating nursing student, this option might have to be considered.
b. Turning a client is the least complex of tasks, so it is the best selection to assign to a PCA.
c. With this option being so general ("returned from an x-ray procedure") it is not a good selection for a PCA. The procedure could have been invasive and complex or it could have been very simple. Since it is unknown, do not choose this option.

d. Discharged clients are typically assigned to licensed persons—preferably an RN if available and an LVN as a second choice. These clients would require reinforcement of education needs and any concerns about discharge plans taken care of.

Test Tips

The important item to note in the situation is what level of personnel is being assigned. Since it is a PCA whose experience level is not disclosed, select the simplest task for assignment.

144. The correct answer is c.

Rationales

a. A right side-lying position is the position of placement *after* a liver biopsy. The question is asking the position during the liver biopsy.

b. This is an incorrect position. Think physiology. If you lie on your left side the liver would tend to move away from the exterior wall of the abdomen and be more difficult to find with a needle stick.

c. This is the correct position. The right arm above the head pulls up the rib cage and makes access to the liver easier. Do this maneuver now to see how it feels. The bed is to be elevated since the client has severe COPD. Low Fowler's position is about a 30-degree elevation. A dorsal recumbent position

is where the client is lying supine on his back, head, and shoulders. The knees may be flexed at 10 to 15 degrees.

d. This option would be appropriate for clients who do not have severe COPD.

Test Tips

Think anatomy. The liver is on the right upper quadrant of the abdomen. The second item to keep a focus on is the time parameter given ("during the procedure," not after the procedure).

145. The correct answer is c.

Rationales

a. Liver studies are monitored for most by-mouth medications. If the child had received oral chelating agents to bind the lead, then this would be the correct answer.

b. Cardiac enzymes are not done to monitor a child for effectiveness of lead poisoning therapy.

c. Since the therapy is of the injection type, the renal studies are to be monitored. *Recall tip:* Creatinine is monitored for evaluation of overall renal function. Creatinine clearance is monitored for evaluation of glomerular filtration rate.

d. Coagulation profiles might be obtained upon the initial diagnosis of lead poisoning and would be monitored only if the baseline results were elevated.

Test Tips

For most injection therapies the renal lab tests are monitored. For oral therapies the liver enzymes ALT and AST are usually monitored.

146. The correct answer is c.

Rationales

   a. Mild depression is not an end behavior for a client with a bipolar disorder.

   b. A mild mania indicates that therapy is not yet effective. The other caution here is the use of the word "mild" without other descriptions of behavior being given. What is meant by mild?

   c. Hypomania is the desired end behavior for a client with a bipolar disorder. To review: the degree of mania determines the degree of depression. The aim of lithium therapy is to control the mania. This is why lithium has the drug classification of mood stabilizer. Clients are typically admitted to units when they are in a manic state. Therefore the end behavior is hypomania, which is somewhere between depression and mania. This is one of a few clinical situations where a "hypo" condition is desired.

   d. This is an incorrect end behavior.

Test Tips

If you have no idea of a correct answer, use the group clustering approach. Cluster options a, b, and d under the umbrella of vague terminology without descriptors. Select the odd man out, hypomania.

147. The correct answer is c.

Rationales

   a. The test results are positive for a client with an immunosuppression problem. A Mantoux test is the same as a purified protein derivative (PPD) test. It is read at the same intervals of 48 and 72 hours.

   b. The second part of this option is correct. The test result is considered positive.

   c. This is the best choice. The client may have other pathology that may contribute to the test result.

   d. The test is not inconclusive because of the suspected AIDS. It is *positive because the client is thought to be immunosuppressed from the AIDS.* Recall that clients who are immunosuppressed have a standard for a smaller induration being positive since their body cannot produce the larger induration. A similar concept is that a low-grade fever is of a concern with these clients because they are unable to develop a high temperature. The test is inconclusive since no other findings are given that might suggest the client has tuberculosis.

Test Tips

You probably narrowed the options to c and d. Careful thinking is as important as careful reading in this question. As option d is written it is an incorrect conclusion to the test result. What you were thinking and maybe reading into the option was "the test is positive because of immunosuppression from the suspected AIDS and is inconclusive. Beware. That is not what is written.

148. The correct answer is b.

Rationales
   a. This action would be last to do since the IV is at a keep open rate.
   b. This is the first task for the nurse to do. Insulin drips have a priority and the fact that a change in the drip rate was ordered within the last 30 minutes further reinforces that this is the initial action to take.
   c. This task would be the second one to complete.
   d. This task would be the third one to complete. Key words are that the blood pressure and output have been maintained on the drip rate for 72 hours. Thus the client and rate are stable.

Test Tips
If you are confused, use the approach of verb and object. For example: option a, check KVO rate; option b, change insulin drip rate; option c, inspect TPN rate and glucose; and option d, evaluate stable dopamine rate. This way your thinking becomes clearer and makes the selection of option b much easier.

149. The correct answer is a.

Rationales
   a. An increased systolic pressure increases or widens the pulse pressure, one of the classic findings of increased intracranial pressure.
   b. An increased diastolic pressure indicates systemic hypertension.
   c. A decreased pulse with a deep breath is a normal physiologic response.
   d. A decreased pulse with suctioning is a normal physiologic response from the stimulation of the vagus nerve. It is called the Valsalva maneuver.

Test Tips
As you read the options, eliminate c and d, which are expected responses. In deciding between the options a and b, if you had no idea of a correct answer, go with what you know. The systolic blood pressure increases and decreases in greater numbers (such as 10 to 15 points at a time) than the diastolic pressure (smaller increments of 2 to 5 points at a time). Therefore it is more likely that the increased systolic pressure is the best answer. Another way to figure this out is to recall what the pressures mean. Systolic pressure is the resistance the heart has to pump against on contraction of the cardiac muscle. Diastolic pressures are the resting pressures of the heart. Therefore it logically follows that the systolic pressure would increase. If intracranial pressure increases it increases the resistance the heart has to pump against.

150. The correct answer is a.

Rationales

  a. This client would be the first to check since the procedure included a blind stick into a major artery. The risk of hemorrhage is the greatest.
  b. This client would be the third one to check. The surgery site is the major artery. However, the procedure included the insertion of a graft and the use of sutures. Thus there is less of a risk for hemorrhage.
  c. This client is the second to check. With a radical neck dissection and laryngectomy the client has minimal risk for aspiration with the permanent opening for the trachea changed to the hole at the client's neck base. If you were thinking of this client being congested you are reading into the question. Yes, this surgery is a threat to the airway, but without more information it does not automatically put the client in a priority to be checked first.
  d. This client would be the last to be checked since no threat exists to the respiratory or cardiovascular systems.

Test Tips
Avoid knee-jerk choices based on the ABCS. Be sure to think through each of the given options.

151. The correct answer is c.

Rationales

  a. This is an expected complaint. The client may have mild difficulty swallowing for as long as 6 to 8 weeks.
  b. This is an expected need for this surgery at this time.
  c. This is of major concern because of the threat of infection.
  d. This is an expected finding that may last 2 to 3 months or longer, depending on the rate of healing.

Test Tips
Key words in the question are "most concern." This guides you to approach the options with the thought that they all are concerns. You have to prioritize them as you read. This type of question is considered a higher level of question and therefore is more difficult.

152. The correct answer is d.

Rationales

  a. This option is too general to be the best option. Where is the edema? The lung? The abdomen? The legs? The face?
  b. Left ventricular hypertrophy is a result of *aortic* valve stenosis or regurgitation.
  c. Hemoptysis is a finding in tuberculosis, pulmonary infarction or embolism, pneumonia, and pulmonary contusion.
  d. When the mitral valve is stenosed or stiff the blood can't get through

to the left ventricle. Therefore it backs up into the left atrium and eventually the lung to cause pulmonary congestion of which dyspnea is a finding.

Test Tips
Think anatomy to get this question correct. Take the time to draw a picture of the heart with the valves. Have your heart anatomically correct by making the right side smaller than the left side (which is the biggest muscle). Then think: the **T**iny side gets the **T**ricuspid valve and the **M**ighty side gets the **Mi**tral valve. Recall that these valves are located between the atria and the ventricle.

153. The correct answer is c.

Rationales
   a. This is an incorrect method, since the medication should not be diluted.
   b. This is an incorrect method, since medication is not to be mixed with formula. In addition you cannot be sure the infant will take all of the formula.
   c. This is a correct method. Medication for thrush in the mouth is to be swished and swallowed. These actions are the closest to this technique for an infant.
   d. This is an incorrect method.

Test Tips
The focus as you read the options is to think of which of these methods is clos-est to "swish and swallow." Also use common sense to eliminate options, especially option d.

154. The correct answer is d.

Rationales
   a. An up-to-date immunization history means that this child would have last gotten the vaccines at age 5 or 6 years as he entered school. The booster should be repeated when this child is around 16 years of age.
   b. Tetanus immune globulin provides immediate protection since it is passive immunity. It is not needed now.
   c. This is an incorrect answer.
   d. This is the correct answer since the child is up to date on immunizations. If the child was not up to date the correct answer would be option c.

Test Tips
Tetanus toxoid, a vaccine, is active immunity. An easy way to remember this is the word "vaccine" has an "a" in it—think active immunity. Immunoglobulins are the opposite—passive immunity. Remember one and say the other is the opposite.

155. The correct answer is d.

Rationales
   a. This statement supports the suspicion of child abuse.
   b. This statement supports the suspicion of child abuse.

c. This statement supports the suspicion of child abuse.
d. This statement does not support the suspicion of child abuse.

Test Tips

The clue to answer this question correctly is to read the question correctly. The way that it is worded mimics an "except" type of question. You may want to reword the question to read: All these factors support a suspicion of child abuse except which option?

156. The correct answer is a.

Rationales

a. Anemia is an indicator that would be seen as the client progresses into chronic renal failure. Erythropoietin is decreased or stopped since the kidney has failed function. Erythropoietin stimulates the bone marrow to produce red blood cells. Epogen can be given to mimic the function of erythropoietin.
b. A client in renal failure usually has hyperkalemia and hyperphosphatemia. The serum sodium will depend on what phase of renal failure the client is in: if in the oliguric phase, hyponatremia occurs from hemodilution; if in the diuretic phase, hypernatremia occurs from hemoconcentration.
c. Diaphoresis is associated with acute conditions. It is not common to see persons walking around with constant diaphoresis.
d. A client in renal failure usually has hypertension from the retention of fluid.

Test Tips

Note that the stem takes you through three events: acute renal failure, hemorrhage, and chronic renal failure. The lab data are given and might have contributed to your confusion. None of them are needed to answer the question. The question is about chronic renal failure.

157. The correct answer is d.

Rationales

a. This option puts words into the client's mouth (that the client thinks of dying).
b. This statement projects the nurse's feeling of discomfort into the client's situation.
c. This statement evades the topic (the client being worried).
d. This is the best statement, since it directly addresses the client's comment of being worried.

Test Tips

If you have no idea of a correct answer, use the matching approach. Match the focus in the stem, "worried" with the option that has that same focus. Select option d.

158. The correct answer is d.

Rationales

a. This sputum is associated with pulmonary edema.
b. This is normal sputum.
c. This is sputum associated with old blood or trauma or dehydration.

d. This is a classic characteristic of sputum with pneumonia. You might wonder how to tell if it is bacterial or viral. This is easily figured out. This sputum is typically from bacterial pneumonia. Viral pneumonia has clear or white, thick sputum.

Test Tips

Did you notice that a similar question was asked before this? Note that the answer was different then since the focus of the question was different, yet the options are all the same. Remember to read with your antennas up and to acknowledge what the question is.

159. The correct answer is b.

Rationales

a. This option is outside of or external to the nurse's control.
b. This is negligence since the nurse omitted or failed to act. Malpractice is different in that the nurse acted and the client was harmed in some manner.
c. This option is outside of or external to the nurse's control.
d. This option is outside of or external to lab results and is more of a courtesy than an obligation to the client.

Test Tips

As you read each option ask yourself what is in the nurse's control and what is external to the nurse's control or obligation.

160. The correct answer is a.

Rationales

a. This is the correct answer, especially if multiple sex partners occur frequently. Other clients at risk for cervical cancer are those pregnant at a young age, those with a history of sexually transmitted diseases, and those with herpes or venereal warts caused by human papillomavirus.
b. Recurrent tuberculosis has no association with cervical cancer.
c. Celibacy is a risk factor for ovarian cancer. Other risk factors for ovarian cancer are seen in clients who are white, nulliparous, infertile, postmenopausal, exposed to asbestos or talc, and who have a family history of ovarian, endometrial, breast, or colorectal cancers.
d. Being elderly and having breast cancer have no association with cervical cancer.

Test Tips

Think anatomy. The cervix can be thought to be the door to the uterus. Then use common sense and ask which of the options would result in stimulation or exposure to the cervix. Of the given options only option a is close, anatomically speaking.

161. The correct answer is a.

Rationales

a. Feeding is directly related to nutrition. The most appropriate method

to do a gross evaluation of a client's nutrition, no matter what the age, is the height and weight.
b. Developmental charts are a more global evaluation of infants. They include interaction and movement observations.
c. This is an incorrect approach to get the most objective information about the infant.
d. This action is indicated if there was an over- or underweight to height situation.

Test Tips
Celiac disease, also called gluten enteropathy, is a disease of unknown etiology. It is characterized by a permanent inability to tolerate gluten, one of the proteins found in wheat, rye, oats, and barley. Findings include steatorrhea, malnutrition, peripheral edema from decreased protein and CHO, bleeding from lack of vitamin K, and anemia from decreased iron, folic acid, and vitamin B_{12}. A gluten-free diet is recommended, with corn, rice, and millet substituted for the above grains.

162. The correct answer is d.

Rationales
a. This is a false statement.
b. This is a partially true statement since endometrial tissue can be found in other areas such as around the fallopian tubes or in the peritoneal cavity. Therefore it is not the best option to answer this question.

c. This is a false statement.
d. This is the only true statement.

Test Tips
Endometriosis is characterized by ectopic growth and function of endometrial tissue. The causes of it are unknown.

163. The correct answer is b.

Rationales
a. The dangers of gonorrhea to the newborn delivered vaginally are ophthalmia neonatorium (also called gonorrheal conjunctivitis), sepsis, and pneumonia.
b. This is the best answer since it focuses on the entire pregnancy.
c. This is incorrect information. Think of this infection as a local infection.
d. This is incorrect information.

Test Tips
If you have no idea of a correct answer, use the group cluster approach. Group options a, c, and d under the umbrella of specific, focused options. The odd man out, option b, is more general. Select option b.

164. The correct answer is c.

Rationales
a. This client would be scheduled third to be visited since the client is 4 days post op without any stated problems.
b. This client would be scheduled second to visit since there is a mother and infant who are 3 days post delivery. Also, there is a specific need for the mother.

c. This client is to be visited first because there are specific physiologic needs.
d. This client would be visited last since no time or other characteristics of the decubiti are given.

Test Tips
If you narrowed the options to b or c, you can use Maslow's hierarchy of needs to put the client with insulin needs (physical needs) before the client with education needs.

165. The correct answer is c.

Rationales
a. This is a false belief that pencils have lead in them. Pencils contain graphite, not lead, even though we call them "lead pencils."
b. There is a risk of lead paint in old apartments. However, avoid reading into the option that the child visits these apartments. Therefore this is not the correct option.
c. This is the correct answer since the house may have lead paint and the child would be spending most of his or her time at home.
d. This building might have lead paint. It is not the best option, since the child is there only three times a week.

Test Tips
For exposure to toxic substances, think not only of the exposure but also of the length of time and the frequency of the exposure.

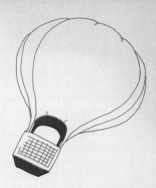

Index

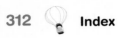